Scottish Borders Library Service

WITHDRAWN
3 4144 0058 994€

D0541294

The Which? Guide to
Asthma and Allergies

About the author

Mark Greener has worked as a pharmacologist in the fields of research and academia, and is now a medical journalist. Mark has contributed to both consumer and specialist publications, including *Health Which?*. He has written numerous articles and several books on the subjects of bioscience, drugs, nutrition, health and the pharmaceutical industry for medical, nursing and consumer magazines worldwide; he is health editor for *Pharmaceutical Times* and was consultant editor on *Pharmaceutical Visions*. For Which? Books he has written *The Which? Guide to Managing Stress* and *Which? Way to Manage Your Time – and Your Life*.

Acknowledgements

The author and publishers would like to thank the following for their helpful comments on the text: Professor Peter Barnes, Dr Harry Brown, Dr Jo Congleton, Dr Bill Frankland, Dr Andrew Menzies-Gow, and Sue Freeman at *Health Which?*.

The Which? Guide to Asthma and Allergies

Mark Greener

 CONSUMERS' ASSOCIATION

SCOTTISH BORDERS LIBRARY SERVICE	
005899469	
CAW	26/11/2004
616.97	£11.99

Which? Books are commissioned by
Consumers' Association and published by
Which? Ltd, 2 Marylebone Road, London NW1 4DF
Email: books@which.net

Distributed by The Penguin Group:
Penguin Books Ltd, 80 Strand, London WC2R 0RL

First edition February 2004

Copyright © 2004 Which? Ltd

British Library Cataloguing in Publication Data
A catalogue record for *The Which? Guide to Asthma and Allergies* is available from the British
Library

ISBN 0 85202 941 1

No part of this publication may be reproduced or transmitted in any form or by any means,
electronically or mechanically, including photocopying, recording or any information storage
or retrieval system, without prior permission in writing from the publisher, nor be otherwise
circulated in any form of binding or cover other than that in which it is published and without
a similar condition being imposed on the subsequent purchaser. This publication is not
included under licences issued by the Copyright Agency.

For a full list of Which? books, please call 0800 252100, access our website at
www.which.net, or write to Which? Books, Freepost, PO Box 44, Hertford SG14 1SH.

Editorial and production: Joanna Bregosz, Alethea Doran
Index: Marie Lorimer
Original cover concept by Sarah Harmer
Cover photograph by SSK-Superstock/A1pix

Typeset by Saxon Graphics Ltd, Derby
Printed and bound in Wales by Creative Print and Design

Contents

★ An asterisk next to the name of an organisation in the text indicates that the contact details can be found in this section

Please note that although this book provides medical information, it is essential that you consult your GP or appropriate health professional for specific advice.

Where brand names of drugs are given, these may be examples only. Other brands may be available from your doctor or pharmacist, while drug brands may change over time.

Introduction

The UK is in the grip of an allergy epidemic. Each spring and summer, for example, some 12 million people endure the misery of hay fever. And the epidemic isn't confined to running noses and streaming eyes. A recent survey by the British Society for Allergy and Clinical Immunology found that more than one in three people in the UK has been diagnosed with at least one allergic disorder some time during their life. Indeed, in the year preceding the survey, over a fifth of adults and children suffered from allergic rhinitis (which includes hay fever), asthma or eczema. What's more, many people have more than one allergic condition. Overall, the UK has one of the highest rates of allergic disease in the world.

A report published in June 2003 by the Royal College of Physicians (RCP) presented similar figures. It noted that the number of people with allergies in the UK has increased nearly threefold over the last 20 years and continues to grow apace. All the allergies discussed in this book have shown a marked increase.

People with allergies show an excessive immune response to substances that most of us find innocuous – and such triggers are all around us. In the UK, pollen, animal dander (dead skin and hair) and microscopic mites in house dust are among the most common causes of allergic reactions. But other triggers include food, latex, antibiotics and other drugs, and bee and wasp stings.

For millions of people, allergies are, fortunately, only a nuisance. But for many, they interfere with normal activities and can, in a few cases, ruin the sufferers' quality of life. Occasionally – for instance, among people with severe asthma or those allergic to peanuts or insect venom – allergies can, tragically, prove fatal.

For all these reasons, allergic conditions impose heavy clinical and economic burdens on the National Health Service (NHS) and on society as a whole. Currently, for example, allergies account for

6 per cent of general practice consultations and 10 per cent of GPs' prescribing budget. Managing allergies in primary care alone, the RCP remarks, costs the NHS £900 million a year.

So – given the human, clinical and economic tolls – you might expect allergy provision on the NHS to be well developed and widely accessible. But, according to the RCP, the service is, in general, poor and fragmented. Its report highlights 'the dearth of NHS services', and points out that management of allergic diseases differs widely across the UK.

In particular, the report notes that the UK lacks a high-quality service able to diagnose and treat allergy. For instance, few general practices and hospitals have the facilities to test whether a person is allergic to a specific allergen (allergic trigger). This means that doctors can't advise patients on the best way to avoid their allergy triggers – instead, people must usually rely on drugs to alleviate the symptoms. And few GPs are specially trained in diagnosing and managing allergies. All this means that people with allergies often have to help themselves: both by learning about their condition so that they can deal confidently with their doctor or nurse and ensure they receive the best treatment, and by changing, where possible, their lifestyle.

The lack of high-quality allergy provision on the NHS in many parts of the UK may help explain the rising interest in complementary and alternative approaches to the diagnosis and treatment of allergies. Understandably, some people consult these therapists because they are dissatisfied with conventional medicine. But – as explained later in this book – there is no convincing scientific evidence that, in general, alternative methods of diagnosis for allergies work. (Indeed, if there were a validated, quick and simple test for allergies, it would be welcomed by the medical profession. Currently, diagnosing the cause of allergies is time-consuming and can give misleading results.) On the other hand, there is compelling scientific evidence that some complementary treatments can alleviate allergic symptoms in some people. However, non-conventional therapies can sometimes be inappropriate, expensive and even harmful. So you need to tread carefully.

Nevertheless, the number of people who consult complementary practitioners demonstrates the growing awareness among allergy sufferers of the importance of taking control of their condition. The key to taking control is to understand why your allergy arises and the steps that you can take to alleviate the symptoms and reduce the likelihood of suffering an exacerbation. To help you understand your condition, this book contains general and specific chapters. Chapter 1 explains the biological basis of allergies. Chapters 2 and 3 examine the common triggers for allergies and the ways in which doctors can diagnose these conditions and identify the cause. Chapter 4 looks at anaphylaxis, a potentially fatal form of allergy. These introductory chapters should provide some background and insights, whatever your allergy.

The next chapters cover specific conditions. Chapters 5 to 7 deal with asthma, its diagnosis and treatment. Chapters 8 to 12 cover some of the other common allergic diseases – rhinitis, conjunctivitis, food allergies and so on. Although you can skip these if, say, you're interested in only asthma, it is worth remembering that, as mentioned earlier, many people have more than one allergic condition. For example, children with eczema commonly react to certain foods. Hay fever can develop into asthma. So it might be worth making sure that you don't also suffer from one of the other allergic diseases.

Finally, Chapter 13 looks at some of the complementary and alternative approaches that have been tried in the diagnosis and treatment of allergies. It examines the scientific evidence, if any exists, for their effectiveness. It unravels some of the misconceptions surrounding these approaches to allergic disease, and offers guidance in an area that can be something of a minefield.

You do not need any medical knowledge to understand the information and explanations in this book. While some technical terms are unavoidable, these are explained in the text and listed in the glossary. The book contains bibliographic references to the scientific papers that formed the basis for its recommendations. There is also a list of non-specialist further reading.

Currently, allergic conditions cannot be cured. But, through a combination of modern medicines, lifestyle changes and, in some cases, complementary and alternative treatments, most people with allergies can live normal, healthy lives.

Chapter 1

Allergies and the immune system SCOTTISH BORDERS COUNCIL

LIBRARY &

INFORMATION SERVICES

The seventeenth-century philosopher Thomas Hobbes famously described life as 'nasty, brutish and short'. This may not always be true of modern times – at least in the developed world. But the world around us remains hostile. For instance, many of the bacteria, viruses, fungi, other micro-organisms and parasites that surround us can cause serious, even fatal, diseases.

Our immune system usually protects us from dangerous micro-organisms. But sometimes the immune system can go awry. And allergies arise when it goes awry in a particular way. This chapter explains how an excessive immune reaction gives rise to allergies.

This explanation involves using some medical terms and, at first sight, the process might seem complex. However, getting to grips with the theory will help you understand the diagnostic techniques and treatments that are discussed in later chapters and help you feel informed when you talk to your doctor or nurse. So it's worth taking some time over. On the other hand, you don't need to follow the arguments outlined here in order to benefit from the practical suggestions in the rest of the book. In this chapter we also look at the roles of genetic and environmental factors in the development of allergies, and address the question of why allergies are becoming more common.

Why we need immunity

It's hard to grasp the number of micro-organisms in our environment. Around 800 to 1,000 bacteria could fit on this full stop. Many biologists, with good reason, consider micro-organisms in general and bacteria in particular to be the most successful form of life on earth. Scientists have found bacteria on the deepest seabeds and the highest mountain, from some 12 km below sea level to 8 km above. Bacteria can even thrive in the water that dribbles through rocks some 3km below ground and in temperatures in excess of 110°C.

Hostile micro-organisms are everywhere. They're in our food. They're in the soil, air and water. They're on our skin, in our airways and inside our guts. One bacterium, *Helicobacter pylori*, which resembles a jelly bean with four-to-six whip-like tails, can even thrive in our highly acidic stomachs. *H pylori* can cause ulcers, dyspepsia and stomach cancer.

New diseases caused by micro-organisms are emerging all the time: over the last decade or so, severe acute respiratory syndrome (SARS), West Nile virus and Ebola were among the new fatal infections to hit the headlines. And each flu season, researchers wonder whether this year's strain will lead to a repeat of the Spanish Flu pandemic of 1918, which killed between 20 million and 40 million people worldwide.[1]

Given the opportunity, many of these potentially dangerous viruses, bacteria and fungi would invade the surrounding tissue from the air in our lungs or the food in our gastrointestinal tracts. And yet, despite the millions of micro-organisms around us, most of us don't normally succumb to them. Our immune systems (helped, of course, by improved public health, vaccinations and antibiotics) keep infections in check.

All organisms have evolved defences against attack from disease-causing micro-organisms – also called pathogens. If they hadn't, evolution would probably have come to an abrupt halt. Even bacteria produce enzymes and other chemicals that counter invasion from pathogens. Plants produce numerous chemicals to protect them from infection. But the most sophisticated and versatile of these defences is the mammalian immune system.

What is immunity?

The word 'immunity' derives from the Latin *immunis*, meaning 'free of a burden'. The basic function of the immune system is to keep us free of the burden of infection. To achieve this, our immune systems identify and destroy invading pathogens. We say that someone is 'immune' after they have been vaccinated against a particular disease. So, for example, the pertussis vaccine confers immunity against whooping cough. Rubella vaccines confer immunity against German measles. The BCG (Bacillus Calmette-Guérin) vaccine makes us immune to tuberculosis (TB).

Once we are immune, we are much less likely to contract a further infection when we encounter that specific pathogen. With some vaccinations, the immunity is virtually total and lasts for life. You only need one BCG vaccination, for example. In other cases, the immunity reduces, but doesn't eliminate, the likelihood of contracting the infection. And sometimes the vaccine's effects can wear off after a number of years. For example, the immunity against tetanus (lockjaw) wears off, so you need a booster every ten years or so.

Obviously, the immune system is a lifesaver – just look what happens when HIV undermines the immune response in people with AIDS, for example. But the system is on a fine biological tightrope. And sometimes it loses its balance.

The so-called 'autoimmune diseases' offer an example of what can happen when the immune system loses its balance. In people with these diseases, the immune system starts destroying healthy tissue. In other words, it loses its ability to distinguish healthy from diseased tissue. In people with rheumatoid arthritis, for instance, the immune system destroys healthy cartilage and bone in and around the joints. In people with type 1 diabetes – the form that usually emerges in childhood – the immune system destroys the cells in the pancreas responsible for producing insulin, a critical hormone. In the case of multiple sclerosis, many neurologists believe that the immune system destroys the myelin sheath that surrounds the nerves. (Myelin 'insulates' the nerves in a similar way as the plastic coating surrounding a wire.) Allergies are not autoimmune diseases. But they arise from a dysfunctional immune system.

Your body cannot predict which infections you will encounter over the course of your life. For this reason, the immune system is able to mount both specific and non-specific reactions. As the name suggests, specific immune responses counter particular micro-organisms. So if you've been exposed to a particular flu strain, your body can mount a specific reaction against that virus. (It is this specific-response function of the immune system that, when it targets an inappropriate substance, causes many allergies.)

But, as flu mutates readily, the immune system might not be able to counter a different strain. (That's why some people – see page 88 – need a flu jab each year. The vaccination formula is changed each year to reflect the strains that experts believe are likely to pose a threat that season.) As we'll see later in this chapter, the specific immune reaction takes time to emerge. So the immune system also contains cells that are relatively non-specific. These respond to a wide range of possible pathogens, including those that you haven't encountered before. The non-specific immune reaction helps to keep an infection in check while the specific response has time to develop. For example, some types of white blood cells engulf the invading micro-organism in an attempt to keep the infection localised in one part of the body. The non-specific immune reaction also leads to a fever. The increased body temperature helps your immune system work more effectively. This non-specificity is very useful – but nevertheless, it might be one factor that contributes to autoimmune diseases: a dysfunctional non-specific reaction can also attack certain healthy cells.

What is allergy?

Essentially, allergies occur when the immune system mounts an excessive response to a specific trigger that most people find innocuous. Scientists call this trigger the 'allergen'. An apt description of the allergic response compares it to the way that 'one well-placed cannon shot at the mountain can start an avalanche of snow'.[2] The allergen is the 'well-placed cannon shot' and the immune reaction is the avalanche. And the patient is 'buried' in the symptoms of asthma, hay fever, eczema and so on. Together, allergic rhinitis (which includes hay fever) and the allergic forms of asthma and eczema are known as the 'atopic diseases' (from the Greek *atpos*, meaning 'out of place'). The reaction is out of place because the trigger, if it didn't cause this allergic reaction, would not pose a threat to the person. (Strictly speaking, 'atopic' means that the person inherits a genetic predispostion to produce antibodies known as IgE – see 'How allergies arise', page 16 – to environmental allergens. Allergies can also arise in people without this genetic predisposition, caused by several mechanisms, which we'll consider elsewhere in this book.) The box below outlines the hallmarks of these three common allergies.

The most common allergic diseases

- **Asthma** (see Chapters 5–7) is caused when the allergen constricts the airways, leading to shortness of breath.
- **Hay fever** (see Chapter 9) arises when the allergen causes inflammation of the lining of the nose, leading to blockage and discharge. These symptoms are also known as 'rhinitis' and, depending on the allergen, can be seasonal or perennial (occur all year round).
- **Eczema** (see Chapter 8) is characterised by red, inflamed skin following exposure to the allergen.

There are numerous possible allergens. For example, some foods, certain drugs – even proteins that leach from the latex in rubber gloves, condoms and medical tubing – can provoke allergies. In most cases the allergen is a protein. So, despite its reputation, airborne pollution (such as car fumes and cigarette smoke) does not directly cause allergies. However, pollution, as well as passive and active smoking, can increase susceptibility to allergens and exacerbate the symptoms. We will look at the common allergens and non-allergic triggers again in the next chapter. In the meantime, for the purposes of the following explanation it is important to remember two key points.

- Firstly, the response is specific for that person and that allergen. The 'avalanche' triggered by the allergen is an example of a specific immune response. For example, most people can stroke a cat or dog without developing a rash. They can vacuum without the house dust starting them wheezing, or walk through the park without grass pollen triggering runny eyes and nose. But people allergic to these allergens find that exposure leads to, for example, eczema, asthma and hay fever respectively. Moreover, hay fever is triggered by different allergens in different people. Not all hay fever sufferers are allergic to grass pollen; some react to fungal spores or tree pollen, for example.

- Secondly, minuscule amounts of allergen can provoke marked immune reactions. Even a trace of peanut in a take-away meal, for example, can set off severe, even potentially fatal, anaphylaxis (see Chapter 4) in susceptible people.

When we talk about allergies, then, we are referring to only those conditions arising from changes in the immune system. Often people may say that they are, or their child is, allergic to certain foods, such as milk, eggs or wheat. This may mean that they develop unpleasant symptoms, such as bloating, after eating these foods. These symptoms shouldn't be dismissed, but, in most cases, they are not allergies – the immune system isn't involved. These are the so-called food intolerances. (We will return to this key distinction in Chapter 11.) Nevertheless, allergic reactions to food can be severe and, even, life-threatening. There is a danger that by using 'allergies' to refer to, say, mild bloating after a glass of milk, people won't take the condition seriously enough when faced with, for example, a potentially fatal peanut allergy.

How allergies arise

As we have seen, allergic reactions are excessive immune responses to specific allergens. To understand how this excessive reaction occurs we need to explore the immune system in a little more depth. Even biologists find the subtleties of the immune system difficult – so you might need to read this section a couple of times. But it will help to make sense of the underlying principles. It will illuminate how allergic diseases emerge, how they can be diagnosed and how drugs (see box on pages 22–3) and other treatments, such as immunotherapy (see box on page 19), work.

While hay fever, asthma and eczema differ in their symptoms, most cases of the atopic forms of these diseases are caused by the same underlying mechanism, outlined in Figure 1 opposite. The 'immune cascade' that leads to the allergic reaction is explained in the following pages.

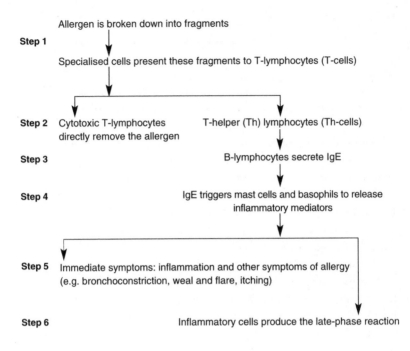

Figure 1   The immune cascade

Step 1

As you probably know, blood contains several different types of cells. Red blood cells (erythrocytes) carry oxygen from the lungs to your tissues and carbon dioxide back to the lungs. Platelets help your blood to clot. And white blood cells are an important part of the immune system and aid the fight against infection. There are several different types of white blood cell. The type we're interested in at this stage of the immune cascade are known as T-lymphocytes, or T-cells.

When you inhale a pathogen or allergen, or it lands on your skin, specialised 'dendritic' cells (mobile cells in the blood, the skin and the lining of the lung) capture and ingest the foreign protein. Enzymes in the dendritic cell break the protein down into small fragments, called peptides. The dendritic cell then moves to the local lymph gland: small swellings that drain lymph (a colourless liquid that bathes cells) and produce some white blood cells. (That's why doctors feel around your neck if they suspect you have an infection.

You have a ring of lymph glands there that can become swollen with cells containing the offending micro-organisms.)

Step 2

The lymph glands are home to numerous T-lymphocytes, including memory T-lymphocytes, which help the body respond to specific pathogens it has encountered before, and cytotoxic T-lymphocytes, which destroy the invading pathogen or the allergen. Dendritic cells bind to and activate another type of T-lymphocyte, the T-helper (Th) cells, which release mediators (chemicals that bring about effects in other cells) that stimulate another group of white blood cells: the B-lymphocytes. We will take another look at Th-lymphocytes when we consider a leading theory explaining why allergies are becoming more common, at the end of this chapter.

B-lymphocytes produce antibodies. Essentially, antibodies allow your immune system to 'remember' which pathogens (or allergens) it has been exposed to. This way the immune system can mount a rapid, effective response the next time you encounter the pathogen.

The first time you are exposed to the pathogen you don't experience any symptoms. But after the first exposure, your immune system is primed ('sensitised'). So when you're exposed to the pathogen again, your body is able to generate the antibodies and mount the immune response much more quickly and to a much greater extent. This is the biological equivalent of being vaccinated. When you encounter the pathogen for the second or subsequent time, your body can rapidly destroy the infection, often before it produces symptoms.

Unfortunately, if you're primed to respond to an allergen – known as 'sensitisation' – you'll develop allergic symptoms, through the mechanism described in Steps 4 and 5 below. As mentioned in Step 4, these reactions are parts of normal responses to 'invaders' – you sneeze whether the trigger is pollen or an infection. You can develop a rash in response to a skin infection, a chemical or an allergen. But in allergic diseases this reaction is targeted against a substance that non-allergic people find innocuous.

Step 3

So, the next time you are exposed to the pathogen (or allergen), B-lymphocytes secrete antibodies. There are several types of

Immunotherapy

Immunotherapy, also called desensitisation, switches off the response to the allergen – the 'immune cascade' – and is effective in seasonal allergic rhinitis (hay fever) and mild seasonal allergic asthma, as well as in allergies to bee and wasp stings. Desensitisation might also be effective against allergies triggered by cat dander and house dust mites, as well as in perennial (year-round) allergic rhinitis. However, a report in 2003 by the Royal College of Physicians[3] suggests that more studies are needed to confirm the benefits of desensitisation in these cases. The report also comments that immunotherapy does not seem to benefit people with non-allergic rhinitis, mild allergic asthma, atopic dermatitis (allergic eczema), chronic urticaria ('hives') or food allergies.

Immunotherapy is relatively expensive for the NHS. So both you and your doctor need to be committed to finishing the course of treatment, which can take several years. For this reason, immunotherapy is used only in severe cases – mainly to treat allergies to wasp and bee venom and for severe hay fever that does not respond to drugs.

During desensitisation the doctor injects increasing amounts of extracts of the allergen below the skin. Once the injections reach the top or 'maintenance' dose, treatment continues at this level, usually for three years. This switches off the 'immune cascade'. The person remains 'desensitised' for several years after the course of treatment ends.

Desensitisation can cause serious side-effects, however. Therefore the doctor will monitor you carefully for at least an hour after each injection and will have resuscitation equipment close at hand. There is a risk – especially in people with both allergic rhinitis and asthma – of suffering severe asthma attacks or anaphylaxis (an extreme allergic reaction – see Chapter 4). This risk is highest during the initial treatment course, although severe reactions can occur at any time. For this reason, immunotherapy is performed only in allergy centres by experienced allergists (doctors who specialise in allergies).

antibody, each with different and specific roles. In people with allergies, the antibody responsible for the symptoms is known as Immunoglobulin E (IgE). We seem to have evolved IgE to help tackle infections by certain types of parasites, in particular the helminths, such as tapeworm.

In allergies, the antibody is specific to the allergen. So, for example, people with allergies to cat dander (dead skin and hair), produce specific IgE against cat dander. Those allergic to grass pollen produce specific IgE against grass pollen, and so on. In general – although there are exceptions to this rule (see Chapter 2) – IgE does not cross-react. This means that people who produce IgE against cat dander don't react to grass pollen, and vice versa. If they are allergic to both, they produce IgE specific to grass pollen and another IgE specific to cat dander. This specificity means that doctors can use a number of tests for IgE to determine whether your symptoms are caused by allergies and to try to define which allergen you are sensitive to. We will examine these tests in Chapter 2.

Step 4

IgE antibodies then bind to a third type of white blood cell: the mast cell. Each mast cell has stores, known as granules, that contain chemicals called inflammatory mediators. As their name suggests, these chemicals trigger and control inflammation. Everyone – allergic or not – knows the symptoms of inflammation. The affected area becomes red, swollen, hot and, usually, painful. It might not be immediately apparent, but inflammation underlies almost all allergic symptoms. In hay fever, for example, the inflammation affects the nose and eyes. And inflammation deep in the lungs is responsible for most cases of asthma.

The antibody's binding triggers the mast cells to degranulate. That is, the granules release their stores of inflammatory mediators. The mast cells also freshly synthesise a number of other inflammatory mediators as a direct response to the antibody's stimulation, which are then released. IgE also binds to basophils, another type of white cell, and triggers the release of yet more inflammatory mediators. These mediators enhance the inflammatory response and cause many of the symptoms of allergy (see Step 5).

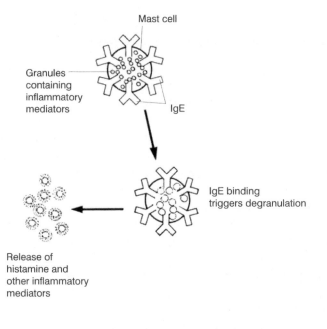

Mast cell

Granules
containing
inflammatory
mediators

IgE

IgE binding
triggers degranulation

Release of
histamine and
other inflammatory
mediators

Adapted from *Immunology Simplified* (OUP 1984)

Figure 2   Antibodies trigger release of inflammatory mediators

Step 5

Histamine is one of the most important inflammatory mediators
released by mast cells. Histamine binds to small proteins, called
receptors, on the surface of other cells in the body. This switches on
specific biological 'machines' inside the cells, producing allergic
symptoms. (Many drugs work by blocking or stimulating receptors
on nerves or muscles – see box overleaf.)

For example, the binding of histamine to receptors on small
blood vessels (capillaries) triggers dilation. This causes the area to
redden. These blood vessels become more leaky. As a result, the
surrounding tissue swells ('oedema'), producing a weal. Histamine
also binds to and stimulates local nerves controlling the diameter of
the surrounding blood vessels, producing a less marked dilation.
Doctors describe this as 'flare'. These effects are, perhaps, most
obvious in the skin: people with eczema develop red, raised weals –
so-called 'weal and flare' (see also 'Urticaria', Chapter 8). Indeed,

How some anti-allergy and asthma drugs work

Some anti-allergy drugs act on the mast cells. **Cromolyns** (such as sodium cromoglycate), 'stabilise' the mast cells, thus preventing the degranulation. **Antihistamines** alleviate allergies by blocking histamine's action.

As explained in Step 5, histamine acts by binding to small proteins (receptors) on the surface of various cells in the body. This switches on specific biological 'machines' inside the cell, which generate the symptoms. Imagine that the receptor is the ignition lock on a car. The cell is the car, and histamine is the key. When the key fits into the lock, the car starts. And when histamine fits into the receptor, the cell's internal 'machines' start and you get the response – the weal and flare, for example. Figure 3 shows how antihistamines prevent histamine's effect on blood vessels.

Now imagine that you have another key. It fits into the ignition, but it doesn't turn. You can't start the car. And while it's in the lock, you

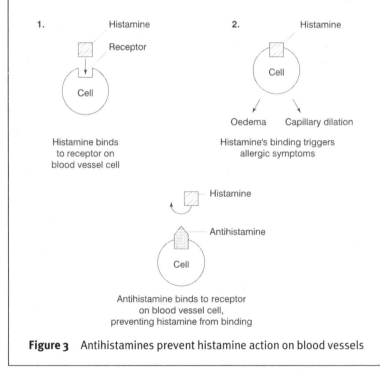

Figure 3 Antihistamines prevent histamine action on blood vessels

obviously can't get the original key in. Antihistamines work in the same way: they sit in the receptor, but they don't activate the cell's internal machinery. Antihistamines stop histamine from binding. In this way they alleviate the symptoms caused by histamine.

Anti-allergy drugs may also target some of the other mediators released by mast cells. For example, montelukast (Singulair) and zafirlukast (Accolate), used to treat asthma (see Chapter 7), block a group of inflammatory mediators called leukotrienes, which potently constrict the bronchi and stimulate mucus secretion. Ongoing research is identifying a plethora of inflammatory mediators responsible for allergic inflammation. And many more drugs acting on specific chemicals are currently being tested.

Steroids – the so-called 'preventers' or anti-inflammatory drugs – are one of the most widely used treatments for inflammation. They are hormones that 'switch off' certain genes in a number of inflammatory cells, such as mast cells, stopping production of inflammatory mediators. Steroids work mainly by crossing the cell membrane that surrounds each cell and binding to receptors. (As described earlier, receptors are small proteins. Most receptors are in the cell membrane, but steroid receptors are inside the cell.)

The complex of receptor and hormone migrates to the cell nucleus, where it interacts with specific sequences on the DNA (the double helix that makes up your genetic blueprint). These sequences switch certain genes on or off. Each gene codes for a protein. The steroid changes the balance of proteins produced by the inflammatory cell, so there are fewer inflammatory mediators produced. Because steroids work at a genetic level, their anti-inflammatory effects can take several hours to emerge.

Some asthma relievers (called **bronchodilators**) relax the muscles around the airways. This eases breathlessness. But, as we'll see in Chapter 7, bronchodilators – in contrast to steroids – don't reduce the inflammation that underlies asthma. Steroids dampen down inflammation, but they act too slowly to alleviate the immediate symptom of asthma: the bronchoconstriction. That's why most people with asthma need to use both bronchodilators and anti-inflammatory drugs.

doctors use the 'weal and flare' reaction to assess the cause of allergies using skin prick and patch tests (see Chapter 3).

When histamine binds to receptors on sensory nerves it produces an intense itch. When it binds to some glands, the person develops a runny nose or eyes. And histamine and other mediators released by mast cells can cause muscles to contract – for example, in the lungs, causing the ring of muscle surrounding the airway to contract. This is one cause of the breathlessness characteristic of asthma.

Doctors describe the symptoms produced by histamine and other rapidly-acting mediators released from mast cells as the 'immediate' or 'classical' allergic reaction. These symptoms develop within 5 to 10 minutes. They wear off after 30 to 60 minutes of exposure to the allergen, as the mast cells' stores of inflammatory mediators are depleted.

Step 6

Some of the inflammatory mediators released by mast cells and basophils 'recruit' several other types of white blood cells into the inflamed area. Once in the inflamed area, these inflammatory cells release a variety of further mediators that maintain the inflammation. They also release enzymes that begin to break down the inflamed tissue. It takes several hours for sufficient cells to reach the inflamed area, so this causes a resurgence of inflammatory symptoms between two and eight hours after the initial exposure to the allergen. This is called the late-phase reaction.

Eventually, however, if you're no longer exposed to the allergen, the inflammation subsides – until you are exposed to it again.

Anaphylaxis

In most cases, the 'immune cascade' described on the previous pages leads to unpleasant and uncomfortable, rather than dangerous, symptoms. But in a few people the immune response is so extreme that they develop anaphylaxis, a severe allergic reaction that can prove fatal. Severe anaphylaxis tends to develop within minutes of exposure to the allergen, and the condition progresses rapidly. This combination of severity and speed makes anaphylaxis especially 'frightening to deal with'.[4]

Fortunately, injecting adrenaline into muscle – which can be done by the person experiencing the attack or by his or her parent or carer – rapidly relieves anaphylaxis. The injection allows time to get to hospital for further treatment. With effective treatment, most people recover completely from anaphylaxis. The symptoms and management of anaphylaxis are dealt with in Chapter 4.

Links between atopic diseases

As you might expect from the immune cascade that underlies many allergies, many atopic people suffer from more than one allergic disease. If the allergen lands on the skin it can trigger eczema. If it sticks in the nose, the person suffers hay fever. If it is inhaled, asthma may result. (That's why many leading specialists, for example, dermatologists and respiratory physicians, call for people with severe allergies to see a doctor specialising in allergic diseases – an allergist. There are, however, too few allergy clinics to meet demand. So people with allergies may need to see, for example, a respiratory specialist as well as a dermatologist, even though the underlying dysfunction in the immune system is the same.)

Many people with allergic asthma also have hay fever. And suffering from allergic eczema as a baby seems to increase the risk of developing asthma or hay fever in later childhood. In one study,[5] for example, 40 children who had been treated as infants for widespread eczema were re-examined at the age of 11 to 13 years. The eczema had disappeared in 18 per cent of the children and in 65 per cent had become less marked as they got older. But 78 and 53 per cent of the children had developed allergic rhinitis (e.g. hay fever) and asthma respectively. Only 20 per cent of those that had eczema as a baby suffered from neither asthma nor eczema in later childhood.

In a study[6] of 1,456 children aged ten years living on the Isle of Wight, almost a fifth (19 per cent) had hay fever, while 23 per cent had rhinitis. Children with rhinitis were more likely to suffer from wheezing – a key symptom of asthma – or from asthma itself. Allergic eczema at four years of age also increased the risk of developing rhinitis at ten years of age. Clearly, then, many atopic people will need to manage more than one condition.

Why do allergies run in families?

Doctors recognised decades ago that allergies tend to run in families. Indeed, the first study showing that a tendency to develop allergies could be inherited was published in 1916. The researchers found that 48 per cent of patients with allergies reported a family history of allergic disease. In contrast, only 14 per cent of allergy-free subjects said that someone in their family suffered from an allergy. Moreover, the researchers reported that 68 per cent of children born to parents who both suffered from allergies developed allergic diseases – compared with 51 per cent with one allergic parent. And they discovered that, as mentioned above, children with allergic asthma also often had hay fever or eczema.

More recent research confirms the strong family association. The Isle of Wight study referred to above found that the ten-year-old children of mothers and fathers with rhinitis were more likely to develop rhinitis themselves. Children of mothers with food allergies were also at increased risk of developing rhinitis.

Children and parents obviously share a large amount of genetic material. Broadly, you get half your genetic material from your mother and half from your father. (This isn't a perfect division. Most cells in your body contain mitochondria, which are responsible for producing energy. Mitochondria contain their own genetic material, which you always inherit from your mother. This is one way in which scientists can track our ancestral lines. But for the purposes of this book, you can consider it a 50:50 split.) So, if you have rhinitis, perhaps your mother, father or both passed on genes that predisposed you to developing the condition.

However, differentiating between environmental and genetic factors can be difficult. In other words, something in the environment shared by the parents and the children could trigger rhinitis in both. So how can we tell whether allergy is in the genes?

One way to determine the relative significance of genes and environment is to examine the risk of developing a condition in identical and non-identical twins. Identical twins are known as 'monozygotic' and non-identical twins as 'dizygotic'. A zygote is a fertilised ovum (egg). So monozygotic means the twins originated from a single (mono) egg that split after fertilisation. Dizygotic means that two ova were released and fertilised. In other words, identical twins have the same genetic profile. Non-identical twins are no more similar genetically than siblings born after separate pregnancies. But, critically (in the vast majority of cases), dizygotic twins are brought up in an identical environment.

Therefore, any differences in the risk of developing a disease between a pair of identical twins are probably due to environmental factors. If a disease were determined solely by genes, identical twins would be equally likely to develop the condition. If a disease were determined solely by lifestyle, the risk of developing the disease in identical twins would be the same as that in non-identical twins brought up in the same environment. The incidence of most diseases falls somewhere between these two extremes. Increasingly, researchers recognise that both 'nature' and 'nurture' contribute to the risk of developing most diseases, although the relative importance varies.

Allergies are no exception. They too seem to arise from an interaction between genes and environment. For example, a study[7] from St George's Hospital Medical School, London, found that monozygotic twins were more likely to share allergies than dizygotic twins.

The researchers estimated that genetic factors accounted for approximately 60 per cent of the difference in IgE levels between the people enrolled in the study. In other words, environmental factors accounted for 40 per cent of the variation in IgE levels. Similarly, a Danish study of twins[8] found that genetic factors accounted for 73 per cent of the risk of developing asthma. So environmental factors accounted for just over a quarter of the risk.

These and many other studies show that genetics is an important factor in determining your risk of developing atopic diseases. Nevertheless, environmental factors are also influential. The risk of developing allergies depends on the complex interaction of environmental and genetic factors.

To appreciate this concept, think about how we learn to speak. We seem to be genetically programmed to learn a language. But whether we learn Swahili or English depends on our environment. Likewise, you might be genetically programmed to develop an allergic disease. But whether you develop allergies or not – and whether you develop eczema, asthma or hay fever – depends on your environment.

This suggests that you may be able to reduce the likelihood of developing some allergies by changing your environment. Doctors call this 'allergen avoidance', and we will look at some lifestyle techniques to reduce your exposure to allergy triggers in the next chapter. In fact, it is the changes in the environment that seem to be responsible for the marked increase in allergies in the industrialised world over the past couple of decades.

Allergies on the increase

Allergies are common in the industrialised world. Very common. A couple of examples underline the point. Firstly, 20.4 per cent of 27,507 children surveyed in the UK suffered from asthma during the year prior to the survey.[9] Furthermore, 18.2 and 16.4 per cent had suffered from allergic rhinoconjunctivitis (hay fever affecting the nose and eyes) and eczema respectively. Secondly, a quarter of British and Australian children under the age of 14 years are asthmatic, while a fifth suffer from eczema.[10]

Over the last 30 years or so, a growing body of evidence has emerged suggesting that allergies are becoming much more common than they were in our parents' and grandparents' generations. For instance, the number of Swedish children suffering from allergic rhinitis, asthma or eczema doubled between 1979 and 1991.[11]

But why are allergies becoming more common? Some researchers comment that the 'striking increase' in allergic disease is not solely a result of improved diagnosis and greater awareness among the general public.[12] We've already seen that genetic factors play a large part in people's susceptibility to allergies – yet genetic changes occur slowly, often over thousands or millions of years, and cannot, therefore, be responsible for the rapid increase in allergic diseases over a few decades. So the increase must be caused by changes in our environment.

Scientists have come up with several explanations to try to account for the rise in allergies. One of the most widely accepted – although it remains somewhat controversial – is known as the 'hygiene hypothesis'. Essentially, this holds that 'a cleaner environment and fewer childhood infections'[12] lie at the root of the increase in atopy.

The hygiene hypothesis

As mentioned at the start of this chapter, your immune system needs to 'learn' to mount specific reactions against potentially dangerous pathogens, such as tuberculosis, flu or measles. So you can think of a rubella vaccine, for example, 'teaching' a person's immune system to protect him or her against German Measles. When a specific reaction goes awry, allergies develop. In other words, in genetically susceptible people the allergen 'teaches' the immune system to mount an inappropriate response against this trigger.

Remember the Th-lymphocytes mentioned in the discussion of the 'immune cascade' (see pages 16–24). Th-lymphocytes, or Th-cells, stimulate B-lymphocytes to produce antibodies. Antibodies allow your immune system to 'remember' which pathogens (or allergens) it has been exposed to. Then the immune system can mount a specific response rapidly the next time you encounter the pathogen – or allergen.

There are two main types of Th-cells: Th_1 and Th_2. These play complementary roles in the battle against infection. Th_1-cells help eradicate, for example, bacterial infections, such as cholera and tuberculosis. Th_2-cells counter parasites, in particular helminths, such as tapeworms, living in the intestines.

You need both a Th_1 and a Th_2 response to survive. But you have a limited number of Th-cells. So the balance between Th_1 and Th_2 depends on the micro-organisms and parasites you're exposed to. If you encounter parasites, especially in early life, the balance will tip towards Th_2. If you're exposed to bacteria, Th_1-cells will predominate. Nevertheless, the response of either Th_1 or Th_2 is more marked in some people than others. And the strength of this response seems to be genetically programmed.

A strong Th_1-cells response has favoured survival when people are exposed to epidemics of infectious diseases. A predominance of Th_2-cells has favoured survival for people exposed to helminths. So, for the population as a whole, it is an evolutionary advantage to have a mixture of people with different responses along the Th_1–Th_2 spectrum. This allows the species to respond to changes in the environment.

Many allergies are caused by a Th_2 response: an increase in the number of Th_2-cells means higher concentrations of the mediators linked to allergic symptoms. And, in addition to this, allergies share several other features with the response to helminth infestation – including IgE production and high levels of certain late-phase mediators in the inflamed tissue. Moreover, helminth infections tend to be common in the less developed parts of the world where allergies are uncommon, and vice versa.[13] So this seems to suggest that if the Th_2 response targets helminth infections it doesn't have enough cells left to induce allergies.

But high levels of Th_2 cells mean fewer Th_1 cells, and vice versa. You can illustrate this by looking at the relationship between rheumatoid arthritis and allergic asthma. (Rheumatoid arthritis is an autoimmune disease, and an excessive Th_1 response seems to contribute to these types of disease.) Allergies, as we have seen, are Th_2 reactions. And people with allergies are less likely to develop rheumatoid arthritis. Correspondingly, those with rheumatoid arthritis are less likely to develop allergies. For instance, one study[14] found that 19 per cent of people without rheumatoid arthritis suffered allergic diseases – this compared with 8 per cent of those with rheumatoid arthritis.

So why has the Th_2 response come to predominate in the West, leading to the allergy epidemic? Until the start of the last century, helminth infections were rife, even in developed countries. And we were much more likely to develop infections during childhood. Today, improved hygiene, vaccination and antibiotics mean that infections are less common. This is obviously, in general, good news. For example, before 1901 in England, diarrhoea accounted for 30 per cent of infant deaths.

But it also means that the immune system of children growing up today does not learn to develop a strong Th_1 response. As a result, the Th_2 arm becomes relatively stronger.[13] But, there are even fewer helminths to tackle. So the Th_2's action isn't directed against parasites. Instead, the Th_2 reaction develops against environmental allergens. So people now mount the immune response their ancestors did against helminths – such as hookworm, threadworm and whipworm – to house dust mites, pollen and cat dander. And we have seen that the tendency towards a strong Th_1 or strong Th_2 response varies between individuals – so it is those people with a strong Th_2 response who may be particularly susceptible to allergies.

The 'hygiene hypothesis' is unlikely to account entirely for the increase in allergy rates, although many researchers regard it as the best theory so far devised. Nevertheless, several other aspects of our Western lifestyle – including air pollution, increases in indoor allergens (especially house dust mites), crèche or nursery care for pre-school children, pre-natal maternal diet and many other factors – may all contribute to the rising number of people with allergies. Clearly, further research is needed to determine the causes of the allergy epidemic.

Chapter summary

The immune system protects us from potentially dangerous micro-organisms. Allergies arise when the specific immune system goes awry. In many cases, this produces an excess of IgE, which leads to the release of inflammatory mediators. These inflammatory mediators cause the symptoms of allergies and are the targets of many of the drugs used to treat hay fever, asthma and other atopic diseases.

The risk of developing allergies depends on the interaction between genetic and environmental factors – and it seems that allergies are becoming more common because of changes in lifestyles in the industrialised world over the past few decades.

Chapter 2

Allergic triggers

As we saw in Chapter 1, people with allergies have an excessive immune response to substances that most of us find innocuous. These triggers can range from food to antibiotics and other drugs (see Chapter 12), latex to wasp venom, and pollen to microscopic mites, to mention a few allergens. This chapter examines the common allergens as well as the main non-allergic triggers that can exacerbate, in particular, asthma, rhinitis and eczema. It also looks at why some people are allergic to, for example, a range of different foods. The tests that may be able to identify which allergen is responsible for your symptoms are dealt with in the next chapter.

Identifying the allergen

The timing of your allergic symptoms can offer some clues to the cause, as the table on page 34 showing pollen seasons suggests – although to be certain you will need to undergo a skin prick test or other assessment (see Chapter 3.) For example, if your hay fever or asthma emerges in early spring it might well be caused by tree pollen. If symptoms arise in late spring or summer, grass and weeds could be responsible. Fungal spores, another common allergen, tend to trigger symptoms during the late summer and autumn. However, more than 20 different moulds in the UK can trigger allergic reactions, and those that occur indoors can cause perennial (year-round) rhinitis and asthma.

Some people react to more than one allergen. People can be allergic to both grass and certain tree pollens, for example. And people with a latex allergy frequently develop allergic symptoms in response to certain foods, including banana, kiwi fruit, avocado and pineapple (see pages 42–3). Many of those allergic to birch pollen also show allergic symptoms when they are exposed to, for example, apple, kiwi fruit, potato and avocado.

This 'cross-reactivity' doesn't contradict the key principle outlined in Chapter 1, that an allergic reaction is specific. In some cases, the person develops specific IgE to more than one allergen. In other cases – such as with birch pollen and apples – the two allergens share a common protein that acts as the trigger. Indeed, some 70 per cent of people allergic to birch pollen may also experience symptoms after consuming, or being in contact with, certain foods.[1] (So, for example, they may develop eczema when they peel potatoes.) This is because birch pollen contains a group of proteins called profilins, which are also found in a number of other plants, including apple, orange and kiwi fruit and raw vegetables such as celery, avocado, potato and tomato. It seems that people who are allergic to birch pollen produce IgE against profilins, so they cross-react to these foods. In other words, they develop allergic symptoms to more than one allergen. Doctors describe chemicals such as profilins, which are present in a number of different allergic triggers, as pan-allergens.

These factors obviously make identifiying the allergic trigger in such cases difficult. Undergoing some of the tests outlined in Chapter 3 is the only way to pinpoint the allergen.

Common allergens

In the UK, the major causes of allergy are pollen, house dust mites and animal dander (dead skin and hair). These and other allergic triggers are discussed below.

Pollen

Grass is the most common cause of pollen-related allergies, as noted in a report in 2003 by the Royal College of Physicians (RCP).[2] Indeed, 95 per cent of people with hay fever are allergic to grass pollen. Levels of grass pollen are high between late May and early August (so, ideally, you should begin treatment to prevent symptoms – see Chapter 9 – a couple of weeks before the start of this period).

The concentrations of grass pollen peak in June and July, especially on warm, dry days with a gentle wind. Levels tend to be highest in the morning and late afternoon. In contrast, grass pollen counts are low on cool, blustery days. As this suggests, both the timing and severity of pollen seasons are influenced by the weather. Indeed, researchers in the UK[3] found that global warming has led to the pollen seasons for birch and other trees beginning earlier.

Pollen at different times of the year	
Month	**Plant source**
March	alder, poplar, elm, yew
April	birch, plane, ash, willow
May	oak, horse chestnut, hornbeam
June	grass, plantain, pine lime
July	grass, nettle, dock, sweet chestnut

Around a quarter of people with hay fever are allergic to birch pollen. (So – as 95 per cent are allergic to grass pollen – obviously, a fair proportion of people with hay fever are allergic to both grass and birch pollen.) Levels of birch pollen peak during April and May. But, as we saw earlier, many people allergic to birch pollen cross-react to other plants, and this means they also exhibit symptoms when exposed to other members of the same botanical family, including alder, hazel and hornbeam. Alder and hazel flower earlier than birch, while hornbeam flowers later. So the hay fever season for these people can be considerably longer than you would expect from the time that the birch pollen is in the air.

Furthermore, the pollen season for many other trees overlaps with that for grass pollen. So some people who believe that grass causes their allergy might, in fact, be allergic to tree pollen. Finally, many weeds – in particular, nettle, plantain and dock, release pollen in late summer and early autumn. So symptoms confined to the autumn might be caused by weeds. And although a number of people believe that they are allergic to oilseed rape, the RCP report mentioned earlier comments that few people are truly allergic to this, and that in fact, in most cases, the adverse reaction seems to follow irritation after exposure to chemicals released by the plants.

Avoiding pollen is, of course, difficult if not impossible. After all, it is borne on the wind. Nevertheless, if you are allergic to pollen there are certain precautions you can take. In particular, it is worth keeping an eye on the predicted levels. The UK is one of the world leaders in monitoring and predicting pollen levels. Currently, 33 sites around Britain produce standardised information that is stored at the central National Pollen Research Unit★ at Worcester's University College. Weather forecasters use these data to offer you some warning of days during which the pollen count is likely to be high. On these days it is worth trying, as far as possible, to stay indoors, especially in the early evening. You could also follow the advice in the box below.

Pollen avoidance

As well as staying in on high-pollen-count days, there are other steps you can take to reduce your exposure to pollen, as follows.

- Keep the windows at home and in your car closed.
- Consider asking a mechanic to fit special filters to your car to reduce the amount of pollen that gets inside. If you're buying a new car, see if you can have these fitted as an optional extra.
- Wear wraparound sunglasses. These prevent the pollen getting into your eyes and triggering conjunctivitis (see Chapter 10).
- Wash your hair regularly. Pollen can stick to your hair.
- Change your clothes after being outside.
- Wash or wipe animals that have been in long grass.
- Avoid grass cutting.
- Avoid camping and picnics.
- Take holidays by the seaside – pollen counts tend to be lower than inland.

House dust mites

It's a very unpleasant thought: your bed and carpets are infested with millions of microscopic creatures that feed on your dead skin cells, fungi, bacteria and organic waste. (The outer layer of your skin – the stratum corneum – is dead. You shed these dead cells continuously). These invisible squatters, one of the most common causes of allergies, are present in incredible numbers. There can be as many as 5,000 house dust mites in a gram of dust. Your mattress may be home to two million mites.

House dust mites are most at home in bedding, soft furnishings and dusty environments – wherever there is plenty of dead skin to feed upon. Dust mites use enzymes (specialised proteins) to digest their feast of dead skin cells. These enzymes accumulate in their faeces. When inhaled, the enzymes in the faeces can trigger the immune response that leads to asthma and rhinitis (and skin exposure can, in some patients, exacerbate eczema). Indeed, when the tribes of New Guinea started using bedsheets the number of cases of asthma rose markedly. The house dust mite, it seems, was to blame.

Precautions against house dust mites

It's impossible to eradicate house dust mites from your home. Using a powerful vacuum cleaner (see box on page 38) sucks up both the mites and the skin cells – but even the most vigorously cleaned house is still home to millions of mites. Nevertheless, it's worth trying the following approaches.

- Wash bed linen above 60°C. This kills the mites.
- Use anti-dust-mite covers (also called anti-allergy covers) for the mattress, duvet and pillows (not everyone finds these effective but they may work for you).
- Because the mites prefer warm temperatures, try turning down the central heating and opening some windows. The increase in insulation over the last 30 years or so means that the air in a typical house is replaced ten times less frequently than in the past.[4]
- Remove furnishings that can harbour dust, such as carpets and thick curtains.
- Avoid clutter. Keep things in cupboards rather than on shelves.
- Wash children's soft toys or put them in the freezer for a day or so. Both will kill dust mites.
- If you are vacuuming a dusty room, try taking an antihistamine beforehand and wearing a mask.
- Get out more. We spend more time than ever indoors, watching TV and so on. Apart from contributing to obesity, this also increases the amount of time that we're in contact with dust mites and other indoor allergens.
- You could try an air purifier – a device that draws air through filters that trap particles (see box opposite)

Improving indoor air quality

Concerns about air quality in the home have led many people with asthma and other allergies to consider buying a dehumidifier, portable air conditioner, ioniser or air purifier, in the hope that this will reduce their symptoms. These devices work in a variety of ways.

- **Dehumidifiers** remove moisture from the air. So they reduce damp and condensation.
- **Air conditioners** extract heat from the home.
- **Ionisers** remove pollutants by sending out negatively charged ions that attract dust and smoke particles. The nearest positively charged surface, such as the floor, walls or furniture, attracts the ions. This collects the dust.
- **Air purifiers** draw air through filters that trap particles.

However, a *Which?* article in 2003[5] comments that these may not necessarily improve asthma symptoms. It notes, for example, that 'there's no conclusive link between the ability of air purifiers to remove pollutants from the air and a reduction in allergy symptoms'.

As a result of this lack of evidence, neither the National Asthma Campaign* nor the British Thoracic Society* recommends that people with asthma should try air purifiers or ionisers. The 'seal of approval' scheme by Allergy UK* endorses several air purifiers, but even this shows only that the devices remove airborne dust mites or cat dander – it doesn't mean that the purifier will improve your symptoms. Indeed, the article notes that other approaches (discussed in the box opposite) can reduce allergen levels.

There is not much you can do to reduce dust mite numbers dramatically, but, in addition to following the suggestions above, you could also try using an acaricidal washing detergent, available from pharmacists. Acaricides are chemicals that kill dust mites. However, there is disagreement about the extent to which they reduce the mite population, and treatment needs to last several months. Research has shown that one acaricide ingredient – disodium octaborate tetrahydrate – lowers dust mite numbers as well as levels of their allergens (the enzymes in their faeces) in carpets and sofas. In one study, the number of live mites in the carpets decreased by 60 per cent in six months. Levels of allergen in the carpets and sofas fell by 63 and 47 per cent respectively.[6] In another study, it was found that the combination of an anti-allergy cover for the mattress and an acaricidal washing detergent reduced mite allergens more than threefold after 18 months. Nonetheless, levels of the allergen remained high.[7]

For further advice on managing a dust mite allergy, contact the National Asthma Campaign.*

Which vacuum?

Regular vacuuming can be part of a wider strategy to minimise reactions to dust mites or pet allergens. Many manufacturers have recognised this and fit some of their models with HEPA (high efficiency particulate air) or S-class filters, which are designed to prevent allergens escaping. As part of its regular tests, *Which?* magazine measures the latest models' ability to retain the most allergens and dust. It has found marked differences between the best and worst machines, so it's important to choose carefully. It's best to buy a cleaner with a HEPA filter. However, *Which?* tests have revealed that some models with HEPA filters were ineffective at retaining allergens. While there's no difference between cylinder and upright types, as a general rule, vacuums with bags might be the better choice because some dust canisters on bagless models can be messy to empty. (Full details of ongoing Which? research can be accessed on Which? Online.*)

Domestic pets

The British are a nation of animal lovers. The UK is home to some 15 million cats and dogs – not to mention numerous fish, birds and horses as well as a menagerie of exotic animals. And many people work with animals, for example in science laboratories, zoos and pet shops. Animals shed particles of dead skin, feather and hair – known as dander – which is highly allergenic. So, not surprisingly, contact with animals commonly causes perennial rhinitis, asthma and other allergies in sensitive people.

And, because animal dander is highly allergenic, owning a pet increases the risk of becoming sensitised and developing allergic reactions. A study in Denmark[8] found that having a cat in the house for over eight years increased the risk of sensitisation to cat allergens more than eightfold. People sensitised to other allergens at the start of the study were more likely to develop an allergy to cats than those who were not. However, there was some good news for canine-lovers – owning a dog did not seem to increase the risk of sensitisation to dogs.

Most people let their pets roam at will. So pet dander can become spread throughout the house. For example, cat dander can form as dust on the floor, pervade soft furnishings and even cling to the walls. It also tends to be very difficult to remove. Even stringent cleaning can fail to make much of a difference – you might need to steam-clean carpets to shift it, for example. Indeed, the allergen can remain in the home for several months even if you re-home the cat.

Understandably, many people allergic to pets are unwilling to get rid of their animals. In any case, even if the house is animal-free, sensitive people can be exposed to animal dander when, for example, other pet owners transport the allergen in their clothing. Such 'second-hand' exposure can be a significant allergic trigger. For instance, children exposed to second-hand cat dander at three months of age were found to be almost 11 times more likely to be sensitised to feline fur at two years of age than those who did not come into contact with the animals.[9] The frequency of the children's wheezing when they didn't have an infection – a hallmark of asthma – doubled.

Managing pet allergies

If you are allergic to animal dander, you may find the following precautions help.

- Wash bed linen above 60°C.
- Wash children's soft toys.
- Keep pets off the beds, sofa and other soft furnishings.
- Avoid feather pillows. Many people allergic to pet dander cross-react to feathers.
- If possible, ask someone who isn't allergic to wash and comb your pet every day. Or do it yourself – but wear a facemask and rubber gloves.
- Vacuum well. But if you are vacuuming a dusty room, try taking an antihistamine beforehand and wear a mask. You could also take an antihistamine and wear a mask if you have no alterative but to come into contact with an animal. Discuss this with your doctor

---

Cockroaches

Cockroaches can trigger allergies, and may be common in inner-city areas. However, cockroach allergy seems to occur more often in North America than Europe. Nevertheless, if you are being tested for sensitivity to various allergens through skin prick testing, for example (see Chapter 3), you might want to make sure that cockroaches are considered as a potential trigger, especially if you live in a dense urban environment.

Fungus

More than 20 moulds – growths containing a web of thin strands of fungi called hyphae – can trigger allergic reactions. And, depending on the species and the environment, fungi release spores (the fungal equivalent of pollen). Some species release spores during warm, dry weather. Others release spores during rain or when it's humid. *Cladosporium* and *Alternaria*, two widespread fungi and common causes of allergies, can release spores throughout the year. These fungi grow on dead organic material (such as decaying leaves), and levels peak during harvesting season, when these fungi can cause severe asthma. Overall, levels of fungal spores peak in the early autumn.

Fungi can also make their home indoors. *Cladosporium* and *Alternaria* can occasionally grow indoors. More commonly, moulds such as *Aspergillus* and *Penicillium* thrive in damp conditions. Just look around your window frames where the condensation collects, or in the bathroom of an old, poorly ventilated house – that dark stain could be mould. Fungi living indoors can cause perennial rhinitis and asthma.

There are various things you can do to reduce your exposure to indoor fungal spores. For example, wipe bathrooms and windows with cleaners containing an antifungal agent. Some paints also come formulated with antifungal agent. Keep rooms dry and well ventilated. In severe cases, you might need to move house to escape the spores.

Bee and wasp venom

Bee or wasp stings are usually just nuisances. But, on rare occasions, a bee or wasp sting can cause the potentially life-threatening anaphylactic reactions discussed in Chapter 4. Not surprisingly, beekeepers and their relatives or neighbours, who are more likely to be stung, are especially vulnerable to developing allergies to bee venom. Wasps, in contrast, seem to strike randomly. In the UK, more people are allergic to wasp than bee venom (presumably because few people live near hives and bees are less likely to sting than wasps).

Broadly, bee and wasp stings cause either 'large local' or systemic (non-localised – that is, affecting the whole body) allergic reactions. Large local reactions, as the name suggests, produce swellings around the sting. The person does not develop symptoms elsewhere in the body. Moreover, large local reactions only rarely develop into anaphylaxis. Nevertheless, these reactions are large. They can involve, for example, the entire forearm.

Systemic reactions to bee and wasp venom usually involve a widespread itchy rash. Less commonly, people may develop conjunctivitis, rhinitis, vomiting or abdominal pain. The reaction may develop into anaphylaxis, which tends to occur within 15 minutes of being stung. People suffering from anaphylaxis typically experience skin reactions followed by a sensation of light-headedness. In some cases, the person faints or develops breathing difficulties. A few people develop only a slight rash, but rapidly collapse and lose consciousness, sometimes without warning. People who experience severe systemic reactions or full-blown anaphylaxis to wasp or bee venom sometimes report a feeling of impending doom.

Venom immunotherapy (see page 19) is highly effective at preventing severe reactions to bee or wasp stings and works in up to 98 per cent of people who have severe systemic reactions.[10] Therefore, people allergic to bee or wasp stings – even those who have experienced only local reactions – should be seen by an allergist (a doctor specialising in the diagnosis and treatment of allergic diseases).

Warning

People who experience systemic reactions may well be at risk of developing anaphylaxis (see Chapter 4). For this reason, everyone who develops systemic symptoms following a bee or wasp sting (or any other trigger) should seek urgent medical attention. If someone develops breathing difficulties and faints, collapses or loses consciousness you should assume that he or she has suffered an anaphylactic reaction. Call 999 and administer, if the person has one, an adrenaline injection. With prompt action most people recover fully from anaphylaxis.

Latex

Latex has been used to manufacture medical equipment since 1888. But fears of infection with HIV, hepatitis and other micro-organisms from blood and tissue fluids led to a marked increase in the use of latex gloves and other medical products during the 1980s and 1990s. Many of the one million people who work in the National Health Service, as well as police officers and fire-fighters dealing with injured people, and also hairdressers and laboratory staff are exposed to latex during the course of their work. And there has been a corresponding rise in the number of people showing allergic reactions to latex. Indeed, latex allergy has been described as 'a global epidemic'.[11]

Disposable medical gloves are the most widely used product containing latex, and are the major source of latex allergens.[11] So people undergoing long-term medical treatment, healthcare workers and scientific personnel are at the highest risk of developing latex allergy. Indeed, between 17 and 36 per cent of healthcare and scientific personnel are allergic to latex.[12] (It appears that people with spina bifida – a congenital problem where the spinal cord and surrounding membranes are exposed outside the body through a gap in the spine – are at particular risk. The reasons for this are not entirely clear, but many people with spina bifida are regularly exposed to latex from an early age, because they tend to need numerous operations, diagnostic tests and examinations.) However, the risk isn't confined to healthcare and scientific staff. For instance, one study[13] found that 18 per cent of hairdressers were allergic to latex.

So why does latex induce allergies? Latex products are made from the sap of the Brazilian rubber tree (*Hervea brasiliensis*). The industrial process used to make gloves and other products – called vulcanisation – alters the proteins' structures. Both the natural and vulcanised proteins can be potent allergens. Furthermore, during manufacture these allergens can leach into the cornstarch powder that latex gloves are coated in to help you get them on.

Skin reactions are the most common sign of a latex allergy. Latex can cause irritation, allergic contact dermatitis (see Chapter 8) or anaphylaxis (see Chapter 4). Irritation, which is not an allergic condition, leads to dry, crusty skin. The irritation resolves when the person is not in contact with latex. As we'll see in Chapter 8, allergic contact dermatitis ranges from a few areas of red rash to cracked weeping skin to (in rare cases) widespread eczema. The itching can be severe and the skin may blister, and in some cases the skin can thicken. Allergic contact dermatitis is especially common in people who also have hay fever, eczema, asthma or another atopic disease.

As mentioned above, allergens can also leach into the cornstarch powder coating latex gloves. You can inhale this powder and it can land on your eyes. So allergic symptoms can also arise in the nose, lungs and eyes.

Obviously, if you use latex gloves at work or are undergoing medical examinations or treatment, and you develop allergic symptoms, you need to know whether latex is the culprit. To see whether latex is likely to be the cause of your symptoms, you will have to undertake an allergy test (see Chapter 3.) The increase in latex allergy has led several manufacturers to produce alternatives to latex so, if you use gloves at work, you should still be able to do your job. If you are allergic to latex, you must ensure that your healthcare professionals know, as you could be in danger of suffering a serious reaction during dental treatment, surgery, vaginal examinations or childbirth.

Many people with a latex allergy are also sensitive to certain foods – especially banana, kiwi fruit, avocado, melon, tomato, potato, chestnut and pineapple. In some cases, people show specific IgE (see Chapter 1) to the food as well as to latex. In others, the person cross-reacts to pan-allergens (see page 33), such as patatin, which is found in, for example, tomato, potato and latex.

Non-allergic triggers

As we have seen, there is a wide range of allergens. But there are also a number of non-allergic triggers that can exacerbate symptoms.

Viral infections
Viral infections are a common asthma trigger – many people find that their allergic asthma deteriorates when they catch a cold, for instance. Described as 'infective asthma', this is covered in Chapter 5.

Smoking
Smoking – including passive smoking – can further impair lung function (see Chapter 5) in people with asthma. (That's another good reason, if you need one, to quit. For advice on how to beat nicotine

addiction, see *The Which? Guide to Managing Stress*.) Nevertheless, many smokers seem unaware that their habit is making their asthma worse. Only half of current smokers attending an emergency department following an exacerbation of asthma admitted that smoking worsens their symptoms.[14]

Passive smoking is also an important non-allergic trigger. In a study[15] of six- to seven-year-olds, smoking by adults in the home was one of the most common risk factors for developing wheezing (a hallmark of asthma), eczema and rhinitis. The researchers suggested that reducing exposure to smoke should improve the quality of life for many children with atopic diseases. Levels of particulate pollution (smoke and soot containing small particles of 2.5–10μm in diameter. A μm is a millionth of a metre) are between two and three times higher in the homes of smokers than in those of non-smokers, and the study found that this indoor pollution contributes to pneumonia and bronchitis in children. Passive smoking also increases the chance that your child will develop symptoms when he or she is exposed to indoor allergens, such as house dust mites and domestic pets.[4]

The increased risk applies to adults too. One study[16] showed that being exposed to passive smoke outside the home for more than five hours a day almost trebled the risk of wheezing. The risk of asthma almost doubled. And women seem especially susceptible to these harmful effects of passive smoking.

Pollution

Many people believe that pollution *causes* asthma and other allergies. This is not strictly true – pollution does not trigger immune reactions such as the IgE response we discussed in Chapter 1. Indeed, asthma and other allergies are becoming more common in the industrialised world, while levels of pollution in those counties are declining.[4] Nevertheless, poor air quality can exacerbate asthma, hay fever and other respiratory diseases. So, for example, people with asthma are more likely to have an attack on days when the level of pollution is high.

During the London Smog of 1952, a mixture of fog, smoke and chemical fumes hung so thickly in the air that people could barely see a few yards in front of them. The smog claimed some 4,000 lives in addition to those normally expected at that time of year – and most of the deaths were from respiratory illnesses. The public outcry led to the 1956 Clean Air Act.

But at least you could see smog. Today's pollutants tend to be almost invisible. Having said that, however, try looking over a major city from a hill on a summer's day. You will see a haze. Or, wash your hair after walking around in a city for a day – the shampoo sometimes runs dark. Both offer some visible evidence of your exposure to pollution.

Pollution seems to exacerbate respiratory diseases by making the lungs more likely to constrict. A study[17] of children aged between 10 and 13 years showed that 45 per cent of those living near a chemical factory showed airway hyper-responsiveness (a measure of the lungs' reactivity – see Chapter 5). This compared with 32 and 33 per cent of children in rural or seaside areas. Moreover, 36 per cent of the children near the factory showed evidence of atopic diseases, compared with 27 and 23 per cent in the rural and seaside groups respectively. Genetic variations are unlikely to account for these differences, so it is probably something in the environment – and pollution is the prime suspect. Pollution could, for example, make attacks of hay fever or asthma more likely, so more children are diagnosed with asthma and hay fever.

Pollution is a complex chemical cocktail, so it's difficult to disentangle the individual and combined effects of the various components. For instance, pollution typically contains some, or all, of the following – any of which could be contributing factors to asthma and rhinitis

- **'Acid air'** is produced through a chemical reaction between light, nitrogen dioxide and sulphur dioxide. The reaction forms tiny clouds containing drops of sulphuric and nitric acid. Eventually, this leads to acid rain. If you have seen pictures of the devastation wrought by acid rain on forests, imagine what it can do to your lungs or nose.
- **Carbon monoxide**, mainly emitted from cars, binds to haemoglobin (a specialised protein in red blood cells). As a result, it interferes with red blood cells' ability to carry oxygen from the lungs to other organs. (This is the reason people can die if they are in an enclosed space with car exhaust fumes.) So you are more likely to feel breathless, exacerbating your

asthma or rhinitis. People with heart disease are especially vulnerable to carbon monoxide's effects, and the gas may also damage developing foetuses. But for many people, cigarette smoke is a far more significant source of carbon monoxide than car emissions. Faulty gas heaters can also release the gas, so if you have a gas heater it is prudent to buy a carbon monoxide alarm, which alerts you if levels increase dangerously. If you live in rented accommodation, your landlord should see that an alarm is installed and that it is regularly checked as well as ensuring the heater is serviced regularly.

- **Nitrogen dioxide**, a gas produced by cars, gas cooking or heating and power stations, irritates the lining of the lungs and nose.

- **Smoke and soot** produced by traffic, power stations and coal fires consists of particles of various sizes. Larger particles get trapped in the upper airways and nose. But particles below 10μm in diameter, and especially those below 2.5μm, seem to pose a specific health hazard. Known as 'particulate pollution', these smaller particles travel deep into the lung where they irritate the delicate lining. Furthermore, smaller particles are often rich in a group of chemicals known as polyaromatic hydrocarbons, linked to some cancers. Diesel engines tend to emit more smoke than petrol engines, and particles from diesel fumes may stick to the surface of pollen, making it more likely to trigger an asthma attack or hay fever.

- **Ozone** is a so-called 'secondary pollutant', produced from the chemical reaction that occurs when light falls on nitrogen dioxide and the group of chemicals known as hydrocarbons. So ozone levels tend to be highest on bright, warm summer days. The ozone layer in the upper atmosphere (the stratosphere) protects the earth from harmful ultraviolet radiation, which can cause cataracts and is linked to some cancers, and can damage crops. (That's why there is so much concern among scientists about the erosion of the ozone layer.) At ground level, however, ozone irritates the nose, lungs, eyes and throat. Ozone levels above 90 parts per billion can trigger breathing problems, including asthma, among vulnerable people and those taking strenuous exercise. Fortunately, levels of ozone seem to be falling in many major cities. London saw a fall in peak levels of

56 per cent between 1976 and the end of the twentieth century.[4]

- **Sulphur dioxide**, a gas produced by power stations, diesel engines and coal fires, was the main cause of the respiratory problems during the smogs. Sulphur dioxide constricts the airways, making breathing difficult, especially in young children. Since the introduction of the Clean Air Act, however, sulphur dioxide levels have generally fallen, although they remain high in some industrial areas.

Clearly, then, it is prudent to take precautions when pollution levels are likely to be high. If you have asthma or hay fever, try to avoid going out when the air quality is poor and do not exercise outdoors on polluted days (this also applies to exercising in front of an open window). You may want to increase your dose of anti-inflammatory drug (see Chapter 7 for details of drug treatments for asthma) on days on which levels of pollen or pollution are likely to be high – this is something you should discuss with your doctor.

Chapter summary

The triggers for allergic reactions range from food to pollen, from latex to wasp venom. Moreover, there are a number of non-allergic triggers that can exacerbate asthma, hay fever and so on. In many cases identifying the allergen (the subject of the next chapter) doesn't make any difference to your treatment – asthma management is basically the same whether you are allergic to cat dander or dust mites. And it is often a counsel of perfection to avoid pollen or a wasp sting. But knowing the allergen might enable you to take some precautions.

Chapter 3

Diagnosing allergy

Around 2,000 years ago, the Roman author and physician Celsus described the four hallmarks of inflammation, which doctors still recognise today: *calor, rubor, dolor* and *tumour* – in other words, heat, redness, pain and swelling. We saw in Chapter 1 how the release of histamine and other inflammatory mediators produces these symptoms. For centuries, these hallmarks and the other symptoms they generate in various parts of the body – such as wheezing in people with asthma or sneezing in hay fever sufferers – were all that doctors had to go on in diagnosing allergy. But heat, redness, pain and swelling can also arise from numerous non-allergic diseases – inflammation is part of the body's general defences. And in many cases it's difficult to link the allergic symptoms with the inflammation. In most cases of asthma, for instance, inflammation occurs deep in the lungs, leading to breathlessness, coughing and so on (see Chapter 5).

Sometimes diagnosis is relatively straightforward. For example, a person with red eyes, stuffy nasal passages, severe sneezing and a watery discharge from the nose probably has hay fever. But these symptoms don't tell you which allergen causes the reaction. Asthma triggered by pollen tends to produce the same symptoms as that induced by dog hair, for example.

Fortunately, doctors today can use several tests to determine whether certain symptoms really are caused by an allergic reaction. The tests may identify the allergic trigger, but it is important to recognise that none of them is infallible. Nevertheless, by using a combination of tests, combined with a careful examination of the symptoms, doctors should be able to pinpoint the cause in most cases. Before embarking on some of these tests you may want to discuss with your doctor whether the results will influence your treatment or whether you will be able to take practicable steps to reduce your exposure to the trigger. Otherwise, the test may not be of practical value.

This chapter looks at some of the general tests doctors use to assess people with allergies. Other tests used to assess lung function in asthma are covered in Chapter 6. Chapter 13 examines the alternative 'allergy tests' – such as hair analysis, cytotoxic food tests and the Vega Test.

An allergy diary

When you consult your doctor for the first time about your suspected allergy, he or she will begin by taking a detailed history of your symptoms. But this often proves difficult in the relatively limited time that a GP has for a consultation. And it's often hard to recall any associations between your activities and your symptoms, which might hint at possible causes. So you could help by keeping a diary noting the following things. (But try to keep the entries short and summarise the key points. The doctor still has limited time.)

- **What** symptoms did you develop? The pattern of symptoms can aid diagnosis. For example, people with food allergies may suffer abdominal pain, bloating, vomiting and diarrhoea after eating the offending food. In other cases, the person has a skin reaction. Wheezing, breathlessness during exercise or waking at night with a cough can be the first sign of asthma.
- **When** did you develop symptoms? Do they occur at a particular time of day, for example? (Some plants release pollen in the evening.) Or at a certain time of year? Is it a year-round problem? Rhinitis – runny irritated nose – may occur for a few weeks if caused by pollen, or year-round if triggered by your cat.
- **How long** did the symptoms last? If the exposure to the allergen rapidly causes symptoms, making the link is relatively simple. Remember, however, that some allergic symptoms can occur many hours after the exposure to the trigger. In up to half the cases of allergy, the main symptoms develop between one and ten hours after exposure[1] – the so-called late-phase reaction (see Chapter 1).
- **How severe** were the symptoms? You could try rating the severity on a scale of zero (no symptoms) to ten (worse symptoms ever), for example.

- **What were you doing** before the symptoms emerged? Were you in the garden? Eating a certain food? Was it a high pollen count or particularly polluted day? Were you using a particular household product? If your symptoms worsen after making the bed or vacuuming, you could be allergic to house dust mites. Furthermore, although the IgE response (see Chapter 1) is specific, some people cross-react. For example, as we saw in Chapter 2, some people allergic to birch pollen also react to food such as apples, potatoes, oranges and tomatoes. Some of those allergic to latex react to banana, avocado and kiwi fruit. Obviously, cross-reactions make it more difficult to identify the allergen – but keeping an accurate record can help to pinpoint any cross-reactivity. It can also help you to avoid exacerbating factors – non-allergic triggers, such as cigarette smoke and pollution – that worsen symptoms.

- You should also note – and certainly need to tell your doctor – if you are taking any **over-the-counter medicines**, such as anti-histamines or steroids. If, for example, over-the-counter steroids take the edge off your eczema, your GP might be able to prescribe a more potent formulation or regimen. It's also important to ensure that your GP and pharmacist know if you are undergoing any complementary therapies for asthma or other conditions.

Your doctor might ask whether you or a close family member are affected by the atopic diseases (hay fever, eczema or asthma). As mentioned in Chapter 1, a strong genetic element interacts with environmental and lifestyle factors to cause most allergic diseases.

The skin prick test

Although it is over 100 years old, and despite newer, high-tech laboratory tests (described later in this chapter), the skin prick test remains the most common and practicable way to diagnose allergy and to try to identify the cause. Indeed, many GP practices now offer skin prick testing, especially for inhaled allergens – such as dust mites, grass pollen and animal dander, for example. In some cases, the doctor might also test for the so-called pan-allergens (see Chapter 2) or for potential occupational triggers. As IgE (see

Chapter 1) circulates around the body in the blood, skin prick tests can detect allergens that might be responsible for asthma or rhinitis, as well as those that cause skin reactions.

During the skin prick test, a doctor (or nurse) puts a drop of solution containing the suspected allergen on your skin, usually on the inside of the forearm, and then uses a lancet or syringe needle to prick the skin. He or she might test four or six possible allergens at a time, and will also use the solution without any allergen as well as a solution of histamine. (The solution without the allergen or histamine is known as the 'vehicle'. A formulation without the active ingredient is also called a placebo: see box on page 200.) These 'negative and positive' controls respectively allow the doctor to check that the test is working correctly. The solution without allergen shouldn't cause any change. In contrast, the histamine solution should provoke a reaction, even in people without any allergies.

It takes several minutes for IgE to trigger the release of histamine from the mast cells and induce the red weal with flare (see Chapter 1). So after 15 minutes or so, the doctor will record any change. A red weal and flare that is more than 2mm in diameter greater than that produced by the solution alone is regarded as an indication that the particular allergen could be responsible for the allergy.

In some cases, the results of a skin prick test are clear-cut. So if someone reports typical symptoms for the suspected allergy and shows a positive reaction on the skin prick test to one or more allergens, it is likely that he or she has an allergy. No typical allergic symptoms and no reaction on the skin prick test means an allergy is unlikely.

Many people, however, fall between these two extremes. Some show a positive result to one or more allergens, but do not report symptoms of allergy. For example, they may misinterpret wheezing on exercise as a sign of being unfit, rather than asthma. Others may exhibit marked allergic symptoms, but test negative on the skin prick test. Many thousands of allergens can cause allergies and it is impossible to test for all of them. Cases that are difficult to identify may be referred to specialists for further investigation.

Although prick tests can offer valuable insights, several factors complicate their interpretation. For one thing, not all allergens rapidly provoke a response. Moreover, eczema and some other skin conditions can mask the reaction. And some over-the-counter or prescription anti-histamines, steroids and other allergy treatments can mask a positive result, and so should not be taken for a few days before a skin prick test. Discuss this with your doctor. You should also avoid any complementary therapies, such as herbal treatments, again for several days before, as some of these contain natural anti-inflammatory agents. You should ensure that the doctor knows about all the drugs and herbal treatments you are taking.

Finally, skin prick tests are not infallible. For example, infants and the elderly are less likely to produce adequate weals to the histamine solution, making the results difficult to interpret. And the tests can sometimes indicate that people have an allergy when they do not, and vice versa. In one study,[2] researchers skin-prick tested children who developed allergic eczema (see Chapter 8) almost immediately after eating beef. The tests detected all children with the beef allergy. But between 10 and 21 per cent showed false positives (i.e. these tests suggested that the children tested were allergic to beef, when they were not), depending on the extract used in the skin prick test. Again, if the doctor believes there is any uncertainty – for example, if the results are ambiguous – you may be referred for specialist tests.

The advantages of skin prick tests are that they are painless – although they might be a bit uncomfortable and a positive reaction may itch – and that side-effects are uncommon. In very rare cases, the person can develop an anaphylactic reaction (see Chapter 4), especially with food allergens. Nevertheless, skin prick tests are one of the simplest and quickest ways to determine whether you really are allergic and which allergen triggers your symptoms.

The patch test

Patch tests are commonly used to diagnose contact dermatitis and allergic eczema (see Chapter 8). They can be used to test for both allergic and non-allergic triggers of dermatitis, such as chemicals. A small amount of the suspected allergen or chemical trigger is placed under a patch, usually on your back. After 48 or 72 hours, the doctor or nurse will look at the area covered by the patch again. Eczema at the site suggests that you are sensitive to that allergen or chemical. Patch testing can also aid the diagnosis of some drug reactions (see Chapter 12) as well as identifying whether you react to components in skin-care products or cosmetics.

Patch testing is highly sensitive, able to discriminate between closely related chemicals. For example, tetrazepam, a muscle relaxant, can cause severe skin reactions. One study[3] showed that patch testing is able to distinguish between tetrazepam and diazepam, which have similar chemical structures. Diazepam patch tests did not induce a reaction in people allergic to tetrazepam.

As with skin prick tests, patch testing rarely causes marked or serious side-effects. On occasion, however, it can trigger a flare of eczema and can cause sensitisation (predispose the person to having an allergic reaction). This means that the person develops allergic eczema for the first time as a result of being tested.

Again, you should not take over-the-counter or prescription anti-histamines, steroids or other allergy treatments before patch testing, as this could affect the results. Furthermore, researchers have noted that different races may vary in their susceptibility to contact dermatitis (see Chapter 8), which could influence the results of patch testing. Black people may be less likely to develop irritant contact dermatitis than Caucasians. Asian people, on the other hand, might be more reactive.[4] Further work is needed, however, to confirm this finding and determine whether the differences matter clinically. In general, though, patch tests are an invaluable means of assessing which allergen causes contact dermatitis. However, they are time-consuming and usually need to be performed in hospital.

Challenge tests

Challenge (also called provocation) tests, as their name suggests, expose the person to the suspected allergen to determine whether he or she experiences symptoms. Challenge tests can be used for the lungs, nose and eyes – for asthma, rhinitis and conjunctivitis respectively. However, these tests can be unpleasant and, on occasion, lead to anaphylaxis (see Chapter 4). For this reason they are performed only in specialist centres, where resuscitation equipment is available. Because of the risk, they tend to be used only when there is no other way to determine whether a particular allergen triggers a reaction. Accidents rarely occur in a carefully controlled hospital setting, and there is probably no better way to determine whether a certain allergen causes your symptoms – for example, when several possible allergens occur simultaneously, such as in people with

Exclusion diets

Exclusion (or 'elimination') diets are used in the diagnosis of food allergy. There are several variants of the exclusion diet. These diets are classified as a type of challenge test, because, in the 'formal' exclusion diet, you are exposed to the suspect food after it has been excluded from your diet from some time – as follows.

- You exclude suspect foods from your diet for five to eight weeks. (This is easy if the suspected trigger is, say, shellfish; rather harder (without potentially putting your health at risk) if it is, for example, dairy products.

- One of the suspect foods is reintroduced, mixed with herbs and oils to disguise the flavour. This is because there is a risk that you could unconsciously influence the results (see 'The placebo effect, page 200). You note the severity and frequency of any symptoms in a diary. The process is repeated for the other suspect foods.

- At some point, the doctor may introduce a placebo – the herbs and oils without the specific allergen. You – and ideally your doctor – do not know whether you have received the placebo or the allergen, a so-called 'double-blind' assessment. If you react to the placebo, the suspect food is unlikely to be the cause of the symptoms.

More commonly, people will follow a less formal exclusion diet. In this case you ban the suspect food from your diet and, if the symptoms abate, you don't reintroduce the suspect food. You record your symptoms before and during the exclusion period. If the symptoms abate the food might be responsible for your symptoms. About ten days' exclusion should usually be enough to pinpoint the 'culprit' food. If the suspicions are wrong, however, finding the culprit can take months.

Another approach is to exclude everything from your diet apart from a few bland foods. Then you gradually reintroduce a normal diet, noting the response as you become reacquainted with various foods. Exclusion and other diets should be performed only under the supervision of a qualified dietician. Your GP can refer you.

possible food and drug allergies (see Chapters 11 and 12 respectively). Challenge tests can also confirm that allergy is no longer a clinical problem, such as when children grow out of some food intolerances or allergies.

Inhalation tests

Doctors may also use inhalation tests, a type of challenge test, to assess a person's response to specific inhaled triggers or allergens. During the test, you sit in a sealed chamber into which the allergen is introduced. You then breathe in the suspected trigger. Should you suffer anaphylactic shock, the doctor can step in with an injection of adrenaline to relieve the symptoms.

These tests may involve histamine or methacholine (see box overleaf) to test for asthma. In other cases, doctors use specific allergens and occupational (workplace) chemicals. For instance, people suspected of having asthma or rhinitis that is triggered by aspirin might inhale a mist of soluble aspirin. Those who are sensitive tend to react within 30 to 60 minutes. (Inhaling the drug is safer than tests where, for example, people take aspirin tablets – it is easy to stop someone breathing in a chemical; rather harder to remove a tablet from the body. Another method of testing for this trigger involves applying aspirin to the inside of the nose; symptoms usually occur after 15 to 30 minutes.)

Inhalation tests for specific triggers have their limitations, however. Unlike skin prick testing, assessing a wide range of possible allergens is impracticable. Moreover, the test environment is somewhat artificial – contact with the allergen is brief rather than prolonged. In an inhalation test the patient would be exposed to an intense burst of pollen, rather than encountering it throughout the season. This could be reflected in the test results. And it's worth remembering that if skin prick tests show that you test positive to, say, dust mites, challenge tests are unlikely to offer any further information that will allow more effective control of the allergy.

Another fundamental problem with inhalation tests using histamine and methacholine (see overleaf) is that almost everyone with twitchy (hyper-responsive) airways – see Chapter 5 – responds to provocation. This does not necessarily mean that the person has asthma or rhinitis. For example, smokers have hyper-reactive bronchi. So while inhalation tests can provide some insights, additional tests may be needed.

Histamine or methacholine challenge

Almost all people with asthma are hypersensitive (show an excessive response) to histamine and methacholine. These are non-allergenic chemicals, which means that healthy people either do not react to them or show only a mild response. This test allows doctors to determine the degree of bronchial hypersensitivity.

In people with asthma, histamine and methacholine act directly on the muscles surrounding the bronchi, causing the airways to contract (this is known as bronchoconstriction – see Chapter 5). Doctors use the other lung function tests (see Chapter 6) to assess the extent of the bronchoconstriction.

Usually, doctors note what dose of histamine or methacholine will cause a 20 per cent reduction in the person's lung function. People with severe asthma show a 20 per cent reduction in their lung function with lower doses of histamine or methacholine than do people with moderate asthma. In turn, people with moderate asthma react at lower doses than people with mild asthma. And people with mild asthma react at lower doses than those without asthma.

There are, however, several problems associated with histamine or methacholine challenge, such as the following.

- Your lung function while at rest, bronchodilator use, respiratory infections, recent acute asthma attacks and the time of day can all influence results.
- Histamine or methacholine challenge is not appropriate for some people – for example, those with an FEV_1 (a measure of lung function – see Chapter 6) less than 70 per cent of the predicted value.
- A few people with asthma show normal responses to histamine or methacholine challenge; conversely, in rare cases people without asthma may respond to the drugs.
- The histamine and methacholine challenge tests cannot necessarily predict symptom severity, variation over the course of the day or peak flow, another measure of lung function (see pages 98–100).

Immunological laboratory tests

Sometimes doctors will use laboratory and other tests to confirm a diagnosis or to determine which allergen triggers your symptoms. For example, you might undergo a chest X-ray if you cough. Asthma doesn't show up on an X-ray – but coughing is a symptom of several respiratory diseases. The doctor can use the X-ray to exclude these as possible causes of the cough.

Another type of test involves the doctor taking a smear of cells from your nose and, under a microscope, counting the number of white blood cells involved in the late allergic phase. Counting these levels helps the doctor differentiate between allergic rhinitis and nasal symptoms arising from non-allergic causes. Infections, hormonal changes, some drugs and alterations in nerve function can cause rhinitis, without you being sensitive to an allergen.[5] In this test the doctor needs to insert a cotton bud into your nose, which can be uncomfortable.

Other laboratory tests measure levels of IgE, specific for a particular allergen, in the blood. The radioallergosorbent test (RAST) and enzyme-linked immunosorbent assay (ELISA) both measure IgE levels. The amount of IgE in blood can influence the severity of symptoms, but there isn't a hard-and-fast relationship between IgE levels and symptom severity.

Furthermore, even laboratory tests are not infallible. For example, many people with brittle asthma (where the condition deteriorates rapidly without warning) show food allergy (see Chapter 11). Skin prick tests and RAST did not always accurately predict the results of a challenge test with the trigger food.[6] In other words, neither test proved to be especially accurate in determining those people in whom food might contribute to their symptoms.

While RAST and ELISA are safe and specific, they are expensive and the results take some time to come through, so they tend not to be widely used, although some private clinics offer them. Nevertheless, these tests help confirm a diagnosis of allergy and the responsible allergen.

There is some evidence that IgE levels in the blood rise before the symptoms reach a level necessary for a diagnosis of allergies, and this is where these types of tests offer an advantage. In one study,[7] scientists measured levels of specific IgE antibodies to food and inhaled allergens, such as pollen, in children under two years of age who were hospitalised for wheezing, a symptom of asthma. Indeed, 40 per cent of these children showed asthma during their early years at school. In particular, showing IgE to wheat, egg white, or inhaled allergens predicted an increased risk of childhood asthma. So detecting these specific IgE antibodies might allow the early diagnosis of asthma. This suggestion, however, awaits confirmation in further studies.

Finally, in cases of suspected anaphylaxis doctors might measure levels of tryptase, one of the mediators contained in mast cell granules (see Chapter 1). Concentrations of this chemical peak about an hour after an anaphylactic reaction, although it might still be detected several hours later. Although this aids the diagnosis of anaphylaxis, doctors – or carers – should not wait for the results of the test before instigating treatment for suspected anaphylaxis (see Chapter 4).

Chapter summary

There is currently no simple, safe and infallible test for allergy or for allergens. But by a careful review of your symptoms and your allergy history, and using some of the general tests reviewed in this chapter, doctors can gain considerable insight into the cause of your symptoms. Following this, they can help devise drug and lifestyle strategies that allow you to live with your allergy.

Chapter 4
Anaphylaxis

King Menes of Egypt died around 2640 BC, after being stung by an insect. The pharaoh's demise seems to be the first recorded report of a death due to anaphylaxis – a severe allergic reaction. The most common triggers for anaphylaxis include food and insect stings as well as some drugs. But in some cases doctors cannot identify the trigger of anaphylaxis.

Today, the tragic deaths of people who develop anaphylaxis following, for example, peanut contamination of a take-away meal, regularly hit the headlines. Sadly, almost all of these deaths could have been prevented by a simple injection.

Anaphylaxis is an extreme allergic reaction. The difference is not in the underlying immunological cause (see Chapter 1) but the severity and location of the symptoms. Anaphylaxis is a more widespread reaction than other allergies. So, where allergic eczema affects the skin, asthma the lungs, and so on, in anaphylaxis several sites around the body are generally affected. (Doctors describe this as a 'systemic reaction'). Some people develop the related 'oral-allergy' syndrome: tingling or itching in their mouth when they ingest a certain food.

Anaphylaxis follows the rapid release of massive amounts of inflammatory mediators from mast cells (see Chapter 1). Often the reaction necessitates treatment in the Accident and Emergency department. While anaphylaxis is always potentially serious, it is not necessarily life-threatening. But even mild symptoms, such as the oral-allergy syndrome, may be a warning sign, so if you experience this, make sure you see your doctor.

This chapter covers the possible triggers of anaphylaxis (sometimes called anaphylactic shock) and describes the symptoms of an attack. It explains the simple medical treatment that could save a life if you or someone near you suffers an anaphylactic reaction. It also offers some suggestions for steps you can take to prevent a further episode if you have had one attack.

Anaphylactic triggers

In most cases of anaphylaxis, the underlying process is that described in Chapter 1. Allergens enter the bloodstream and the binding of specific IgE antibodies triggers the release of mediators from mast cells. In a few cases, however, mast cells can release mediators without IgE binding. This is known as an anaphylactoid reaction (see also the 'pseudoallergic' reactions to drugs – Chapter 12).

For instance, aspirin and related medicines, called non-steroidal anti-inflammatory drugs (NSAIDS) – which include ibuprofen (such as Brufen, Nurofen and Hedex) and diclofenac (Voltarol, Diclomax and Motifene) – are among the agents that can cause anaphylactoid reactions. Radiocontrast agents – drugs that are injected to help X-rays and other imaging systems visualise tissue – can also trigger the release of mast cell mediators, without involving IgE. Researchers do not fully understand the mechanisms through which these and other substances trigger anaphylactoid reactions. But the treatment and management of anaphylactoid reactions is the same as for anaphylaxis.

Since anaphylaxis is an extreme allergic reaction, it probably won't come as a surprise to learn that many of the substances and allergens with which we are in daily contact can trigger this reaction in susceptible people. But the most common causes of anaphylaxis are foods[1] – including peanuts, tree nuts (for example, Brazils), fish, eggs and latex. (Chapter 11 covers food allergy and intolerance.)

Medicines might be the most common triggers of *severe* anaphylaxis. (Chapter 12 discusses drug-induced allergies in more detail.) Indeed, in one UK study[2] medicines accounted for 62 per cent of cases of anaphylaxis that necessitated admission to hospital. Food and insect stings accounted for 15 and 11 per cent respectively of admissions for anaphylaxis.

Exercise is sometimes linked to anaphylaxis. The risk seems to be highest with vigorous aerobic exercise, such as running, playing tennis, dancing, riding a bike or skiing. In most cases, the condition is linked to an allergen – usually certain foods, such as shellfish, alcohol, fruit, wheat, celery and milk.[3] Sometimes, exercise seems to have been the sole factor, but it's likely that in most such cases doctors were simply unable to identify the trigger. However, how food allergens and exercise interact to cause anaphylaxis isn't clear.

How common is anaphylaxis?

Gaining an accurate estimate of the number of people who suffer from anaphylaxis is difficult. For one thing, doctors and patients can confuse anaphylaxis and severe asthma (see below). Some researchers also believe that anaphylaxis can be confused with a heart attack, especially in older people. But the evidence suggests that anaphylaxis, while not common, isn't exactly rare either.

For example, researchers[4] reviewed the number of cases of anaphylaxis dealt with in an Accident and Emergency department. Based on this, they estimated that one person in every 3,500 – or roughly 0.3 per cent of the population – have anaphylactic attacks outside of hospital. So, given that the UK population is around 59 million, almost 17,000 people are at risk of anaphylaxis.

But the true number of cases may be higher than indicated by this study. Firstly, the analysis included only cases that reached hospital – so it didn't take into account milder attacks. And, as the study was performed in an Accident and Emergency department, it didn't capture those cases of anaphylaxis arising in hospital among people receiving drugs, for instance. Other research[5] suggests that the figures may be much higher – for example, estimating that around 1 per cent of children and 3 per cent of adults develop anaphylaxis and other systemic reactions to insect venom.

Despite these uncertainties about the precise statistics, there seems to be little doubt that anaphylaxis is becoming more common – in line with the increase in other atopic diseases. It is, after all, the severe end of an allergy spectrum.

Symptoms of anaphylaxis

Anaphylaxis is essentially an extreme reaction to inflammatory mediators (see Chapter 1). Because these mediators cause tissues to swell – in the lungs, lips, tongue and larynx (voice box) – and the muscle of the lung to contract, people who develop anaphylaxis, especially those with asthma, can experience breathing difficulties. This is why severe anaphylaxis is sometimes mistaken for acute severe asthma. A report in 2003 by The Royal College of Physicians[6] notes that many fatal anaphylactic reactions are recorded on the death certificates and medical records as acute severe asthma.

As we saw in Chapter 1, the release of inflammatory mediators from mast cells dilates blood vessels. If this happens throughout your body ('systemically') your blood pressure can fall to dangerously low levels. (Your blood pressure is partly determined by the diameter of your blood vessels. If the blood vessels suddenly dilate, the pressure falls.) This fall in blood pressure – called hypotension – can lead to fainting, collapse or loss of consciousness.

A wide range of symptoms can emerge during anaphylaxis, including:

- cardiovascular: low blood pressure, shock, collapse, increased heart rate
- eyes: eyelid swelling, tear production
- gastrointestinal tract: nausea and vomiting, diarrhoea, abdominal cramps or discomfort
- mouth: itching or a metallic taste, swelling of the lips, face, tongue and throat
- nose: congestion, sneezing, swelling
- respiratory tract: wheezing, bronchoconstriction (tightening of the airways), acute asthma attacks, choking, throat tightness
- skin: rash, urticaria ('hives'), erythema (patchy redness of the skin), flushing, itching.

As mentioned, these symptoms can vary in severity. Some people, before developing anaphylaxis, experience only a tingling or itching in the mouth, or a localised rash, in response to the allergen. But as mentioned earlier, such symptoms can be a warning that you are at increased risk of developing a more serious reaction when you encounter the trigger again. So you should always seek medical attention in these circumstances.

Not everyone develops every symptom in the above list during every anaphylactic attack. The exact pattern of symptoms depends, in part, on the area of the body that is exposed to the trigger. For example, insect venom and injected drugs rapidly reach the bloodstream. So a marked fall in blood pressure and shock tends to dominate anaphylactic attacks caused by these triggers. The pattern of symptoms may also depend on the person's age. Children with anaphylaxis due to insect venom usually develop urticaria (a red, itchy rash) and angioedema (swelling of the lips and face), whereas adults tend to develop airway obstruction or hypotension.[5]

On the other hand, food, obviously, comes into contact with the mouth and throat. So food triggers tend to cause swelling of the larynx as well as angioedema. In serious cases, a person who develops anaphylaxis in response to a food trigger may experience severe difficulty breathing.

In general, the symptoms of anaphylaxis start between a few minutes and two hours after contact with the trigger. But on rare occasions anaphylaxis can occur several hours later. Moreover, the symptoms can recur. For instance, between 20 and 30 per cent of people who develop anaphylaxis induced by foods experience a recurrence of symptoms between one and eight hours after the initial reaction.[7] As a rule of thumb, though, the worse the reaction, the more rapidly the symptoms begin. So severe anaphylaxis tends to develop within minutes of exposure to the allergen and progresses rapidly. However, in some severe cases of food anaphylaxis symptoms may not start for up to an hour after eating.

The speed of anaphylactic attacks is one reason they are so frightening and potentially deadly. The person can become overwhelmed by the reaction before he or she has the chance to take appropriate action. So it is very important that everyone in the family, as well as work colleagues, knows how to administer the adrenaline injection (see below).

In the event of emergency

If someone with an allergy develops breathing difficulties and either faints, collapses or loses consciousness it is worth assuming that they have suffered an anaphylactic reaction. Seek medical attention immediately. Don't wait. Call 999 and administer the adrenaline injection (see overleaf).

Treatment of anaphylaxis

Doctors in the seventeenth century noted that soldiers' asthma improved after they were injured in battle. This improvement probably resulted from a surge in adrenaline, a hormone secreted in response to stress and injury. Adrenaline raises the heart and pulse rate, increases the blood pressure and opens the airways. These reactions help prepare your body to deal with stressful events by helping you stand your ground or run away. Biologists describe this as the 'fight-or-flight' reflex. So the surge in adrenaline following injury opened the soldiers' airways, thereby alleviating the bronchoconstriction that characterises asthma.

Today, doctors prescribe adrenaline (which is also called epinephrine) for anaphylaxis and other severe allergic reactions, such as brittle asthma (where the condition deteriorates rapidly without warning). As we've seen, during anaphylaxis the blood vessels dilate and leak, the bronchial tissues swell, the muscles surrounding the bronchi contract and the blood pressure drops, which can cause choking and collapse. Adrenaline acts quickly to constrict the blood vessels and stimulate the heartbeat, countering the fall in blood pressure; it relaxes muscles in the lungs to improve breathing; and helps stop the swelling. In other words, adrenaline counters the changes induced by the surge of inflammatory mediators. As such, adrenaline injections are lifesavers. They give the person time to get to hospital, where doctors can treat the anaphylaxis with a number of other drugs.

In hospital, the person may receive oxygen and an antihistamine injection. In mild cases, oral antihistamines could be enough to alleviate the symptoms. People who continue to deteriorate may be given a drip or a nebulised bronchodilator (see page 138). For people who have asthma and in some other cases an injection of a corticosteroid may be given, although its effect can take several hours to emerge. (See Chapter 7 for more details about these treatments.)

If you or someone in your family is at risk of anaphylaxis, then, it is essential that you carry an adrenaline 'pen' at all times. You could also leave adrenaline pens in strategic places at home, in the office, or in the car. Make sure that your family and workmates know where the pens are and how to administer the adrenaline – as described below, it's not especially difficult. The person at risk should also wear a MedicAlert bracelet (contact the MedicAlert Foundation* for more information) so that healthcare professionals are aware of the possibility of anaphylaxis and the type of sensitivities, such as to penicillin (see pages 194–5), if he or she collapses.

The adrenaline pen contains a spring-activated concealed needle that can deliver a dose of adrenaline rapidly and accurately. In essence, you simply jab the pen into muscle, usually the thigh. The pen automatically delivers the shot of adrenaline. Your doctor or nurse will show you how to use the pen, but it is very simple. The injection is a low dose of adrenaline but it may cause a few side-effects, such as an increased heart rate. Remember that with prompt action most people recover fully from anaphylaxis.

It's also important to remember that adrenaline's effects may wear off after five to ten minutes. As a result, the injection may need to be repeated. So if you live more than ten minutes from hospital make sure you have more than one pen. Furthermore, adrenaline has a relatively short shelf-life. Make sure you get a new supply before the expiry date. (The expiry date will be on the packaging.)

The first time you have an anaphylactic reaction, you should be referred to an allergist – a specialist in allergies. The allergist may consider immunotherapy (see page 19), which switches off the 'immune cascade'. This treatment can be especially effective if the anaphylaxis is triggered by insect venom and in some anaphylactoid reactions. Venom immunotherapy has been found to work in up to 98 per cent of people who experience severe systemic (non-localised) allergic reactions.[5]

Preventing an anaphylactic attack

The first, and obvious, way to prevent an attack is to avoid the trigger of anaphylaxis. So, if you are allergic to a food, it is essential to read labels carefully and ask questions about ingredients in restaurants, including take-away outlets. (Peanuts may sometimes be described as 'groundnuts' or 'arachis' – so be careful.) You might need to press manufacturers as well as restaurant and supermarket staff for detailed information about the composition of the food they supply. Remember that some allergic trigger foods may be present in minute quantities – too small to be identified on the packaging. It might be worth phoning a restaurant in advance.

Shopping for food for a person with a food allergy can be time-consuming and difficult, but if you are in any doubt, don't risk it. (See Chapter 11 for more about managing food allergies.) It's also crucial to warn teachers, babysitters and other carers if your child is at risk of anaphylaxis, and also to make sure they know how to administer the adrenaline injections.

You can work with your specialist or GP to help you develop a crisis plan, which you can pin up at home, carry in your pocket and hand out to teachers, friends' parents, relatives, work colleagues and so on. The Anaphylaxis Campaign★ offers further advice and support about living with the risk of an anaphylactic reaction.

But to avoid the trigger, you obviously need to know what the allergen is. The allergist might use a skin prick test or an immunological laboratory test, which can help you identify the cause. If an anaphylactic reaction was caused by a drug, you might undergo a challenge test. Although this type of test can be associated with some risk, this may be outweighed by the benefits of knowing what drug you need to avoid. You should discuss the risks and benefits with your doctor. These diagnostic tests are covered in Chapter 3.

The allergist can also help you develop a self-management plan to reduce both the number and severity of anaphylactic reactions. For example, a management plan assessed in one study[8] included advice on avoiding exposure and self-treatment in case the person inadvertently consumes the allergen. The plan also offered detailed advice about understanding labels, dealing with unlabelled food, eating out, travelling abroad and so on. Subjects also received a written treatment plan that described the action to take for mild, moderate, and severe reactions: such as when to use antihistamines alone and when to use the adrenaline injection. The researchers found that only 15 per cent of people with a nut allergy had a further reaction when they followed this self-management plan developed with a specialist. They estimated that about half of these people would probably have had a reaction if they tried to avoid nuts but had no advice from an allergist.

In this study, most of the reactions that occurred among people following a management plan were mild and needed treatment with, at most, oral antihistamine. This suggests that developing and sticking to a management plan is one of the most effective strategies you can take to avoid anaphylaxis. You should discuss this with your doctor.

A relatively new treatment for anaphylaxis sets an antibody against an antibody. The treatment involves a gentically engineered ('monoclonal') antibody against IgE. This antibody binds to and neutralises the IgE, thereby reducing the risk of further attacks. However, the monoclonal antibody needs to be given by injection once a month.

Chapter summary

Anaphylaxis – essentially, an extreme allergic reaction – is associated with a number of symptoms that can vary in severity and may be life-threatening. But, whatever the severity, you should always seek medical attention if you develop symptoms that might herald anaphylaxis. If someone with an allergy develops breathing difficulties and either faints, collapses or loses consciousness, call 999 and administer the adrenaline injection. With prompt action most people recover fully from anaphylaxis. After the first anaphylactic attack, you should always obtain advice from a specialist and ensure that you identify the cause of the reaction, if possible. You should also ensure that you know the steps to take to minimise the risk of a recurrence. It isn't always easy to avoid the trigger, but by taking sensible precautions you should be able to significantly reduce your risk of suffering an anaphylactic reaction.

Chapter 5

An introduction to asthma

The earliest mention of the cluster of symptoms we now call asthma is made in the Egyptian Ebers Papyrus, written some 3,500 years ago. The word 'asthma' – meaning 'laboured breathing' – appears in Homer's *Iliad*, written about the ninth century BC. Some 500 years later, the group of Greek physicians writing under the name Hippocrates first used 'asthma' to describe the disease we recognise today. But asthma treatments concocted by Roman and Greek physicians, which included owls' blood in wine, owed more to magic than medicine. Nevertheless, some herbal treatments (see also Chapter 13) might have acted as bronchodilators (opening up the airways) and so alleviated the laboured breathing.

The Spanish doctor Moses Maimonides seems to have been the first to write a book on asthma, while physician to the Sultan Saladin in AD 1190. Maimonides noted that asthma was characterised by sudden, unpredictable bouts of breathlessness. His treatments included copious amounts of hot chicken soup and sexual abstinence. He also had the humility to admit he lacked a 'magic cure'. And a cure still eludes clinicians and researchers today.

The understanding of asthma took a large step forward when physicians in the seventeenth and eighteenth centuries recognised that asthma arose following constriction of the bronchi (the airways in the lung). One doctor called asthma the 'epilepsy of the lungs', reflecting the attacks' sudden, unpredictable nature. As we'll see in Chapter 6, people with asthma today can monitor their lung function using peak flow meters. These measurements reflect the extent of the bronchial constriction, allowing you to detect any deterioration in airflow and take steps to prevent a severe attack.

Today, doctors recognise that most – but not all – cases of asthma arise from inflammation in the lungs. Swollen tissue and increased mucus production leads to narrowing and blocking of the airways, which inhibits the flow of air through the lungs. In most cases, this is a result of an allergic reaction – in other words the changes in the lung follow activation of the 'immune cascade' described in Chapter 1.

Asthma varies widely. Many people develop the hallmark symptoms: coughing, breathlessness and wheezing. But some people with mild asthma may only cough. Some people endure severe, debilitating attacks that can end in hospitalisation or even death. Others have only mild, intermittent attacks. Indeed, asthma isn't really a single disease – it's more a constellation of symptoms that arise from a number of causes.

Modern treatment of asthma follows guidelines that take a 'stepped care' approach, whereby the dose of drugs is prescribed according to symptom severity, monitored by daily lung function tests, as part of a self-management plan. Management of the condition is covered in Chapter 6; asthma drugs are dealt with in Chapter 7. To help with the initial diagnosis and treatment of your asthma you should keep a symptoms diary – noting, for example, when your symptoms occur, how long they last, their severity and what you were doing when they occurred. See 'An allergy diary', on pages 49–50, for guidance.

This chapter examines the different causes and forms of asthma. But before that we need to understand the basics of the lungs' structure and function. First, we will take a look at the symptoms of asthma.

The symptoms of asthma

Not everyone with asthma experiences all the symptoms character-istic of the disease. For instance, in children and in people with mild asthma, coughing might be the main or only symptom. In addition, there are some particular signs to watch for in children (see below). But the following symptoms are typical of the condition:

- shortness of breath
- wheezing
- chest tightness
- coughing
- feeling congested or coughing small amounts of very sticky phlegm that is difficult to clear.

An acute asthma attack is characterised by the following symptoms:

- difficulty breathing and shortness of breath, even when sitting down
- rapid breathing (hyperventilation)
- increased heart rate – partly because an asthma attack can be terrifying
- a feeling of suffocation.

See pages 107–9 for advice on what to do in the event of an acute asthma attack.

Asthma in children

Below is a summary of some of the signs of childhood asthma. But diagnosing asthma in children can be difficult. The diagnostic tests (see Chapter 6) can be hard for children to perform, and many of the possible symptoms of asthma in children can also arise from other causes (such as croup, for example – see Chapter 6. And mucus dripping from the nose into the mouth is a common cause of coughing among children.) As mentioned above, coughing might be the main or only symptom. For example, in one US study[1] it was found that 'mirth' – that is, laughter plus excitement – triggered asthma symptoms in 32 per cent of children with asthma (laughter seemed more prone to trigger asthma symptoms than excitement). And in these cases, coughing was the predominant symptom.

Moreover, about a third of children experience at least one wheezing episode during their first two years of life, usually following a respiratory viral infection. (See 'Infective asthma', on pages 86–9). Most of these cases are mild. After a few days the wheezing begins to lessen and after around two weeks the child returns to health. Many children never experience another wheezing episode. So doctors are understandably reluctant to diagnose asthma after a single episode of wheezing.

The possible symptoms of childhood asthma include:

- repeated attacks of troublesome coughs or wheezing
- a persistent, dry, irritating cough – which may be the only symptom
- wheezing or coughing that disturbs sleep
- wheezing or coughing between colds. Healthy children tend to cough for a few days when they suffer a cold
- shortness of breath after exercise or exertion.

Inside our lungs

Unless something goes wrong, we rarely think about breathing. It's one of those bodily functions, like the heartbeat, that carries on without conscious control. And it's remarkably reliable. Each minute we take about 12 breaths. And we do this hour after hour, day after day, month after month – for some 70 or more years. Respiration is highly effective at moving a large amount of air. Even at rest, about 0.75 litres of air move in and out of our lungs with each breath.

The lungs (see Figure 4) exchange toxic carbon dioxide for life-giving oxygen, which we need for cellular respiration and metabolism. Without oxygen, our cells cannot repair damage or divide. To meet the body's considerable demands for oxygen, the lungs have evolved into one of the largest organs in our bodies. Each lung weighs about 0.45 kg (although as the left lung lies over the heart it is slightly smaller than the right lung). The right lung is made up of three lobes and the left lung of two lobes. They don't expand fully each time you take a breath but, fully expanded, an adult's lungs hold about six litres of air.

The lungs are spongy and fragile. So they are encased in the bony ribcage and protected underneath by a thick muscular sheet, known as the diaphragm. As we'll see later, the diaphragm also plays an important role in respiration. The intercostal muscles, between each rib, aid breathing and offer further protection. Between the ribs and the lungs are two membranes – the pleura. These slide over each other when you breathe in (inhale) and out (exhale). Pleurisy arises when these membranes become inflamed, following, for example, a viral infection.

When you inhale, air moves in through your mouth and nose. Inhaled air then flows down through your throat and into your windpipe – also called the trachea. The windpipe, which is about 10–12 cm long and about 2 cm wide, is protected from crushing by rings of cartilage (rather like the way plastic rings protect a vacuum-cleaner hose). The air is warmed as it travels. Cold air can trigger asthmatic symptoms. In some cases cold air is enough to cause the bronchi to contract even in the absence of any inflammation – this is one factor contributing to exercise-induced asthma (see pages 79–82).

The trachea then divides into two airways called the major bronchi, one supplying each lung. Rather like the branches of a tree, the major bronchi divide some 10 to 25 times into some 20,000 to 80,000 smaller bronchioles – each about 0.5 mm in diameter. These end in the alveoli, little air sacs that look rather like cauliflower florets.

This arrangement crams the vast surface area needed for oxygen transfer into a relatively small space inside the lungs. The 300 million alveoli contained in the lungs would, if spread out, cover the surface of a tennis court. The alveoli are very thin – only a few cells thick. They are covered on the air side in a thin layer of moisture, which dissolves the oxygen. On the other side of the alveoli's surface is a network of tiny blood vessels, known as capillaries. This arrangement allows red blood cells to exchange waste carbon dioxide for oxygen (see box below).

The exchange of gases

- Oxygen from air that has been breathed in dissolves in the fluid covering the alveoli, crosses the thin layer of cells and is taken up by the haemoglobin in red blood cells (erythrocytes). Haemoglobin is a specialised protein that contains four atoms of iron, each capable of binding an atom of oxygen. (That's why low-iron diets are one cause of anaemia, a disease that compromises your blood's ability to carry oxygen. This can make you feel breathless.) Haemoglobin increases the amount of oxygen the blood is able to carry some seventy-fold.

- At the same time, other red blood cells release unwanted carbon dioxide, which moves across the alveoli into the air in the lung. This is expelled when you exhale.

- In the meantime, the oxygen-rich blood is carried from the lungs into the left side of the heart. From here the blood is pumped around the body.

- Once the red cells have delivered their load of oxygen to cells in the rest of the body, they pick up carbon dioxide and return to the right side of the heart. Haemoglobin carries only about 10 per cent of the carbon dioxide produced by the body. About 85 per cent of the carbon dioxide released by your tissues combines with water in the blood. At the alveoli it converts back into carbon dioxide and water and is released. The remainder of the carbon dioxide travels dissolved in the blood.

- The whole process begins again.

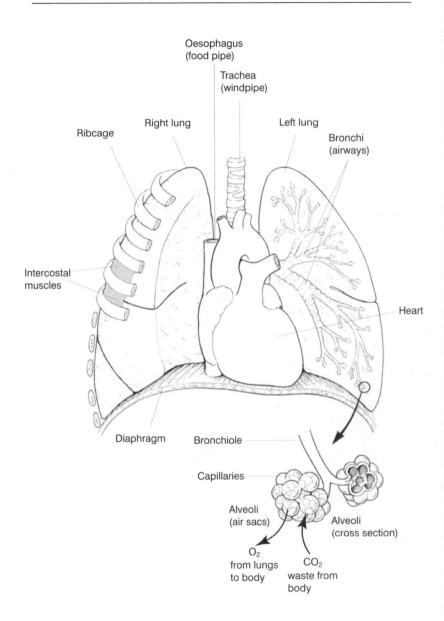

Figure 4   The structure of the lungs

When it's relaxed, your diaphragm curves upwards – rather like a dome. When you breathe in, your diaphragm contracts and flattens. At the same time, the intercostal muscles between the ribs contact and shorten, pulling the ribcage up and out. This draws air into the lungs. The diaphragm and the intercostals then relax and the lungs return to their resting size. This expels the carbon-dioxide-rich air as you breathe out.

The body's control of respiration is very complex. But, in essence, respiration is controlled by an area at the base of the brain known as the medulla, which acts like a thermostat. Receptors in the carotid artery – one of the blood vessels running up the neck – measure levels of oxygen and carbon dioxide in the blood. Nerves pass this information to the medulla. When levels of carbon dioxide rise or levels of oxygen fall, the brain signals to the diaphragm and intercostal muscles to increase the respiration rate. Similarly, when levels of carbon dioxide fall or levels of oxygen rise, the brain signals to the diaphragm and intercostal muscles to decrease the respiration rate. This fine control allows the rate of respiration to adapt to the body's needs. So, when you run for a bus the medulla increases your respiration rate. In contrast, when you rest your respiration rate slows.

The lungs' defence system

Each day, between 10,000 and 13,000 litres of air move in and out of a person's lungs. As we saw in Chapters 1 and 2, the air around us is rich with potentially disease-causing micro-organisms – viruses, bacteria and fungi – as well as aeroallergens such as pollen and irritants including pollution. And these environmental hazards hitch a lift on the respiratory airflow – each breath carries particles, bacteria, viruses, fungi and pollutants deep inside the lungs. So, not surprisingly, our lungs have evolved elaborate defences against these potential invaders.

The nostrils form the first line of defence. They contain hairs that trap large particles and stop them from entering the respiratory tract. (This is an important point: although we talk of allergic rhinitis – inflammation of the nose – and allergic asthma as different diseases, they affect the same organ – the respiratory tract, which begins in the nose and ends in the lungs – and are, in many cases, driven by the same immunological changes. In other words, allergic asthma and allergic rhinitis are symptoms of the same underlying immunological pattern. That's why so many people suffer from both conditions).

Further down the bronchi, smaller particles become trapped in sticky mucus. The mucus is moved by tiny hairs (called cilia) on cells lining the airways. The cilia waft the trapped particles up into the mouth and you swallow the mucus, which is destroyed by enzymes and acid in your stomach. Uncontrolled asthma can damage this 'mucociliary escalator', which may leave you more vulnerable to respiratory infections. Moreover, in some cases infections can trigger asthma (see pages 86–9), so it is very important to ensure that, if you are vulnerable, you have your yearly flu jab.

Bronchioles offer the second line of defence. Bronchioles are flexible tubes surrounded by a ring of muscle. When this muscle contracts, it squeezes and narrows the airway – a process called bronchoconstriction, or bronchospasm. This prevents particles penetrating into the delicate alveoli. In other words, bronchoconstriction is a normal and healthy part of the lungs' defences. (This is why smoking, for example, can trigger bronchoconstriction in people without asthma – we saw in Chapter 2 that smoking is a significant non-allergic trigger).

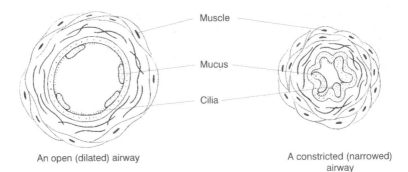

An open (dilated) airway   A constricted (narrowed) airway

Figure 5   Open and narrowed airways

Variations on the asthma theme

In the remainder of this chapter, we'll look at some of the variations on the asthma theme. As mentioned earlier, allergic asthma is the most common form of the condition, but the symptoms of asthma may also arise from non-allergic causes. Furthermore, in some cases, non-allergic causes can make allergic asthma worse.

Allergic asthma

In people with allergic asthma, the inflammation in the airway lining, arising from the allergen-triggered 'immune cascade' we saw in Chapter 1, leads to bronchoconstriction. Bronchoconstriction narrows the airways, limiting the amount of air flowing in and out of the lung. This causes the hallmark symptoms of asthma – wheezing, coughing, and breathlessness – and can result in an acute asthma attack.

In addition, white blood cells involved in the late-phase allergic reaction (see Chapter 1) release chemical mediators that damage the delicate lining of the bronchioles. These late-phase mediators also increase mucus secretion that is more difficult to clear and leave the bronchi of people suffering from allergic asthma excessively sensitive or 'twitchy'. Doctors describe this as 'airway hyper-responsiveness'. This hyper-responsiveness may cause people with allergic asthma to react excessively to non-allergic factors such as cold, heat, air pollutants and infections. In some people, these factors may lead to bronchoconstriction following exposure to lower levels of the allergen than would otherwise trigger an attack.

Initially, the inflammation and symptoms of an allergic asthma attack are reversible – either of their own accord or following treatment. However, prolonged allergic inflammation can irreparably damage the lungs. The walls of the bronchioles become scarred and the delicate cilia are destroyed. Over time, the airway wall thickens (mainly because the amount of muscle increases) and the number of mucus-secreting glands increases. Indeed, among people who die from asthma, the airway wall can be between 50 and 300 per cent thicker than in non-asthmatics.[2] Even in people with asthma who don't die from the disease, the wall can still be between 10 and 100 per cent thicker than in healthy lungs. Moreover, as a result of the increase in the number of glands, the ends of the bronchi can become blocked with sticky mucus plugs. Doctors describe the combination of these structural changes as 'remodelling'.

Because remodelling further reduces the airway diameter in people with allergic asthma, an even smaller amount of airway constriction will produce the same amount of airflow impediment. But there is also some evidence that, in people with allergic asthma, the number of muscle cells around the airway also increases, by between 50 and more than 200 per cent.[2] As a result, remodelling makes a severe attack more likely – especially as the lungs are hypersensitive. In severe cases, the combination of profound bronchoconstriction and increased mucus production can completely block the airways. As a result, airflow stops and, in extreme cases, the person may suffocate (known as 'status asthmaticus').

Doctors still have much to learn about remodelling and just why some people show these changes while others do not. And numerous other questions also remain. The subtle differences between the immune systems of healthy people and those with allergic asthma are not fully understood. Moreover, doctors and scientists need to better understand the way in which genetic factors influence the risk of developing asthma. Some researchers believe that genetic factors could explain why some people with asthma are prone to suffering from nocturnal symptoms (see below), for example. Allergic asthma is the subject of intense research and many of these questions should be resolved over the next decade or so.

Nocturnal asthma

Many people with allergic asthma find that their wheezing and other symptoms are worse at night and early in the morning – a condition known as nocturnal asthma. Indeed, one large study[3] showed that around two-thirds of people with asthma suffer nocturnal symptoms. And this can disturb sleep. In this study, 75 per cent of people with asthma woke at least one night per week, 64 per cent woke at least three nights per week and 39 per cent were disturbed by their asthma every night.

Another study[4] found that about 11 per cent of children aged two to five years habitually snored. Such children were four times more likely to cough during the night and more than twice as likely to suffer from asthma. Among the children studied, 42 per cent who snored also had asthma compared with 26 per cent who did not snore. Quite why asthma is linked to snoring isn't clear. Asthma can make breathing more difficult, which may induce snoring. Alternatively, snoring may allow allergen-laden mucus from the upper airway to enter the lungs.

Not surprisingly, night-time symptoms can leave people sleepy, irritable and tired the following day. This increases the risk of accidents – tiredness can lead to road crashes, for example – and can contribute to stress. Performance at work, college and school may also suffer. Children with asthma often show impaired concentration compared with their school peers, and the effect is especially marked if symptoms are poorly controlled (see Chapter 6 for asthma management) – but children with asthma who are affected by nocturnal symptoms tend to show poorer performance and worse behaviour than those whose symptoms are confined to the daytime.

Many chronic diseases feel worse in the still of the night, when there is little to take your mind off things. Nevertheless, there are several biological reasons why allergic asthma tends to deteriorate in the small hours. Most importantly, the diameter of the bronchioles does not remain constant throughout the day: lung function – how effectively and efficiently your lungs perform (see Chapter 6) peaks around 4pm and reaches a trough around 4am.[5] This pattern, known as diurnal variation, affects everyone – even people without asthma. But in people with allergic asthma, this normal variation is particularly exaggerated. Typically, the average diurnal variation is 8 per cent in healthy people compared with 51 per cent among asthmatics.[3] The late phase of an allergic asthma attack can exacerbate this diurnal variation.

Nocturnal asthma can also be caused by non-allergic triggers. For instance, one study[6] found that exposure to moderate-to-heavy tobacco smoke in the environment – passive smoking, in other words – increased the risk of nocturnal asthma symptoms among children almost threefold.

Many people with asthma experience their most severe chest tightness, lung function and wheezing in the morning when they get up. This seems to reflect the combination of narrower bronchi and increased physical activity. This narrowing is reflected in a decline in the morning peak flow reading (a measure of lung fuction). Doctors call this effect the 'morning dip'.

Nocturnal asthma is a warning signal that allergic asthma may be poorly controlled. Indeed, 53 per cent of deaths from asthma occur during the night.[3] People suffering from nocturnal asthma are more likely to have severe asthma and poor lung function. Yet despite nocturnal asthma being a common, treatable phenomenon (see Chapter 7), many people regard night-time symptoms as a burden they have to live with, even though it may undermine their quality of life. But you shouldn't ignore nocturnal asthma. If you are experiencing these symptoms, make an appointment to see your GP. Nocturnal symptoms are one of the strongest indicators that your treatment may need to be revised.

Exercise-induced asthma

Exercise is good for you, but it is also a common asthma trigger. Indeed, exercise has been shown to be the most common trigger for chronic (persistent) asthma in children.[7] A combination of exercise, hyperventilation (panting) and cold air causes bronchoconstriction in many people with allergic asthma. However, in others exercise is the main, or only, trigger. These people suffer from 'exercise-induced asthma', a non-allergic condition. In these people the FEV1 – a measure of lung function (see Chapter 6) – is normal at rest.

When you participate in exercise, your heart rate rises and your muscles demand more oxygen. As we saw earlier in this chapter, your respiration rate increases to meet the increased demand. Initially, the bronchi dilate (widen) to allow more air into the lungs. In healthy people the bronchi stay open to maintain the greater air flow into the lungs. But in people with exercise-induced asthma the bronchi then constrict. This bronchoconstriction can cause feelings of chest pain as well as breathlessness, coughing and wheezing. Exercise-induced symptoms usually emerge between 5 and 15 minutes after the person starts physical exertion.[8]

In some cases, the asthma might improve on continuing the exercise. During exercise, the body produces a natural hormone, adrenaline, which dilates the bronchi. (We saw in Chapter 4 how adrenaline is used to treat anaphylaxis and brittle asthma.) So as adrenaline levels in the bloodstream rise, symptoms are relieved. Most people recover from exercise-induced asthma within about 20 to 60 minutes, although a few develop a late-phase reaction between 3 and 13 hours later.

Several factors increase the likelihood of developing exercise-related symptoms. For example, cold, dry air is far more likely to provoke an asthma attack than warm, humid air. This may be one reason why some people with asthma find that weather conditions affect their symptoms.

Nevertheless, the cause of exercise-induced symptoms is one area that requires further investigation by scientists. For instance, some researchers believe that cold, dry air increases water loss from the lungs. All animals narrow their bronchi to prevent the lungs from drying out in these environmental conditions; as a result, the airway muscles contract. But among people with exercise-induced asthma the narrowing may be excessive. Other scientists believe the airways may narrow as a result of the cooling followed by rapid re-warming that occurs as a person breathes in and out with an increased respiratory rate. Yet others argue that alterations in immune function (although these seem to be distinct from the IgE-based immunological changes that underlie allergic asthma, as described in Chapter 1) could play a role.

Diagnosing exercise-induced asthma presents something of a problem. Are the symptoms simply an indication that the person is unfit? Is the breathlessness and chest pain a sign of heart disease rather than asthma? Is a child reluctant to take part in sport because he or she suffers from asthma or because of a lack of interest? For these reasons, exercise-induced asthma may go unrecognised and untreated. In some cases, doctors need to measure lung function while patients exercise to determine whether the symptoms are actually caused by asthma.

However, the patterns of symptoms do offer a clue as to whether exercise-induced asthma might be the correct diagnosis. For example:

- children with exercise-induced asthma tend to cough, wheeze and complain of chest pains soon after starting exercise. The symptoms get worse for a few minutes and last for about half an hour

- some children with exercise-induced asthma report suffering from stomach aches
- some children with asthma may avoid sport to prevent symptoms developing. So if your child suddenly loses interest in sport, it might be worth checking whether he or she is experiencing asthma symptoms
- breathlessness that seems excessive compared to the intensity of the exercise may indicate asthma
- older children and adults may develop a 'locker room cough' following physical activity
- you may feel 'out of shape' despite exercising.

If you think that you or your child might suffer from exercise-induced asthma, it's time to consult your doctor or asthma nurse.

Management of exercise-induced asthma

Modern medicines mean that there is no reason why people with asthma should not take part in sport as fully as people without these symptoms. Indeed, many successful athletes have asthma. For example, an Irish study of 305 collegiate athletes[9] found that 24 per cent had a history of asthma. Indeed, other researchers suggest that between 11 and 50 per cent of athletes suffer exercise-induced asthma, triggered by hyperventilation. They also found that, among recreational exercisers, 19 per cent showed airway hyper-responsiveness, while 66 per cent showed asthma on peak flow measurements.[10] So there's no reason why, with effective treatment and by following the suggestions in the box overleaf, asthmatics can't participate in sport.

Indeed, the all-round health benefits of regular exercise are undeniable. Furthermore, some children who do not take part in games may become socially isolated. They can lose confidence, which means they may be less able to fit in with their peers or cope with an asthma attack. As mentioned, drugs can help reduce the risk of an attack while exercising. When taken between 15 and 20 minutes before starting exercise, short-acting beta$_2$-agonists (bronchodilators, or 'relievers') often prevent symptoms. Some other drugs that can be effective in exercise-induced asthma are discussed in Chapter 7.

However, it is important to remember that, for example, a drug that worked in preventing asthma while you played cricket during a warm July afternoon may not work for a cross-country run on a cold, crisp January morning. If symptoms persist you could discuss with your doctor or asthma nurse combining drugs, such as sodium cromoglycate (sometimes spelled cromoglicate, brand names Cromogen, Intal) or nedocromil sodium (Tilade) with a long-acting beta$_2$-agonist. This combination should prevent almost all cases of exercise-induced asthma. Indeed, if you still develop symptoms while using these drugs the cause of your asthma may be another trigger altogether. Finally, if you are a competition-level athlete and are concerned that your medication may show up on drugs tests, check with the Ethics and Anti-doping Directorate.* Most inhaled asthma medications are allowed by sports governing bodies.

How to exercise safely

- Carry your inhaler with you while you exercise or leave it where it is easily accessible (e.g. poolside or touch-line).
- If you begin to wheeze and cough, stop and use your bronchodilator (see Chapter 7).
- If possible, avoid exercise on cold, dry days.
- Exercise in short bursts.
- Exercise using just your arms or legs is less likely to trigger an attack than exercise using both.
- Improve your physical fitness.
- Perform adequate warm-up exercises.
- Cover your mouth and nose.

Some exercises are more likely to provoke asthma than others:

- running tends to trigger asthma more frequently than indoor exercises
- winter sports – skiing and ice skating – are difficult for many people with asthma
- cycling, cross-country skiing and basketball are more likely to cause an asthma attack
- swimming and gymnastics are less likely to provoke symptoms.

Aspirin-induced asthma

In some people, aspirin and related medicines, known as the non-steroidal anti-inflammatory drugs (NSAIDs) – for example, ibuprofen (e.g. Brufen, Nurofen, Hedex) and diclofenac (e.g. Voltarol, Diclomax, Motifene) can lead to asthma symptoms. These drugs are examples of chemicals known as salicylates. Salicylates are also found in some foods (see Chapter 11). In some cases, salicylates are the only trigger for the symptoms. In others, salicylates exacerbate allergic asthma (see below). They can also trigger or exacerbate rhinitis.

Many people with symptoms triggered by salicylates show other characteristics in addition to asthma – for example, most people with aspirin-induced asthma also suffer from chronic hay fever and sinusitis (inflammation of a nasal sinus, a cavity in the nose). Some develop growths inside the nose, called polyps. Doctors may need to perform a challenge test (see Chapter 3) to confirm whether aspirin and related chemicals can trigger or exacerbate your symptoms.

Why some people develop asthma and rhinitis when they are exposed to aspirin is not fully understood, but it probably isn't an IgE-mediated immune reaction (as described in Chapter 1). The following is a possible explanation. Aspirin and other NSAIDs block production of certain prostaglandins (mediators of pain and inflammation) by cells. An enzyme called cyclo-oxygenase creates prostaglandins from a group of fats in the membrane of your cells. NSAIDs block this enzyme, which relieves ache and swelling. This blocking of the enzyme can, however, also stimulate the production of another group of mediators, called the leukotrienes, that trigger bronchoconstriction.

Doctors cannot accurately predict which people with allergic asthma will be aspirin-sensitive. So the safest approach is to avoid exposure to salicylates as far as possible if you suffer from allergic asthma or have developed breathlessness or a blocked nose when taking aspirin, other NSAIDs or salicylates in the past. This means avoiding aspirin and related drugs, as either tablets or creams. Even the tiny amounts absorbed through the skin can be enough to trigger an attack in particularly sensitive people. If you need an 'over-the-counter' painkiller you should try paracetamol and you should tell the pharmacist first. You should also take care to avoid foods that contain salicylates (see Chapter 11). People with aspirin-induced asthma may also cross-react to the dye tartrazine (E102) – see page 185.

Asthma triggered by other drugs

Although the risks associated with aspirin are the best known, some other drugs, most notably the beta-blockers, can trigger broncho-constriction in some people. Doctors prescribe beta-blockers to treat a variety of conditions, including high blood pressure (hyper-tension), some anxiety symptoms and glaucoma. They act in the opposite way from $beta_2$-agonists (relievers, or bronchodilators, which cause the airway to relax). Beta-blockers cause the airways to narrow. In healthy people, this narrowing does not cause any respi-ratory symptoms. In vulnerable people with asthma, however, beta-blockers can provoke an asthma attack and, occasionally, prove fatal. Fortunately, alternative drugs can be prescribed for high blood pressure, anxiety-associated tremor and glaucoma.

Occupational asthma

A report in 2003 by the Royal College of Physicians[11] comments that about one in ten cases of asthma in the UK arises from allergens and other chemicals people encounter at work. In some people – although the proportions are unclear – asthma arises because of sensitisation to allergens found only in the workplace. In other cases, exposure to irritant chemicals at work provokes or exacerbates allergic asthma. (Strictly speaking, the former is called 'occupational asthma' and the latter is called 'work-related asthma'. However, for the purposes of the following discussion we will use 'occupational asthma' to describe both.) And sometimes inhaled irritants can trigger bronchoconstriction in people who do not otherwise suffer from asthma. Occupational asthma is more common in manual jobs; about three-quarters of the reported cases occur in men, and people are diagnosed at an average of 43 years.

Often, the person also develops rhinitis (see Chapter 9) and conjunctivitis (see Chapter 10). Occupational rhinitis can be defined as an 'episodic, work-related occurrence of sneezing, nasal discharge, and nasal obstruction'.[12] This condition can develop independently of asthma and, again, can be either allergic or non-allergic. Substances in the workplace can also trigger skin reactions, such as allergic eczema and contact dermatitis (see Chapter 8).

Occupational asthma was first noted among grain workers in the eighteenth century. Today, we know that some 300 substances in the workplace can cause or exacerbate asthma. But the Royal College of Physicians report mentioned above notes that about a dozen chemicals cause around three-quarters of occupational asthma cases in the UK. The diisocyanates – highly reactive chemicals used to make some foams and plastics, urethane coatings in paints and certain adhesives – seem to be the worst culprits. Diisocyanates have a sharp, pungent odour, and inhaling large amounts can produce a number of unpleasant symptoms, such as nausea, headache, coughing, respiratory irritation, and shortness of breath – even in healthy people. So diisocyanates can cause asthma-like symptoms by directly irritating the lungs.

In some cases, people develop antibodies (see Chapter 1) against diisocyanates. As we saw in Chapter 1, once a person is sensitised, the effect of any trigger is magnified enormously. So very low levels of diisocyanates can produce a serious asthma attack in sensitised people. Moreover, the effects of diisocyanates can persist for many years. For example, respiratory symptoms and airway hyper-responsiveness induced by toluene diisocyanate can persist in people who had not been exposed to the chemical for more than a decade.[13]

Numerous other substances can trigger occupational asthma, including enzymes, latex (see Chapter 2) flour and grain, wood dust and electronic solder fume. In some cases, these are allergic-based reactions. For example, it was found that bakery workers were 22 times more likely to test positive to occupational allergens, such as wheat flour.[14] Other research has shown that inhaled food allergens could play a major role in at least 1 per cent of cases of asthma in adults.[15] Clearly, occupational asthma is a common and potentially serious issue for workers and employers.

If you think that you may suffer from occupational asthma, look out for the three key characteristics (see box overleaf). Do not rely on memory – keep a diary and note where and when your symptoms occur and how severe they are. And remember that you may use some of the same chemicals that could trigger your asthma at home and at work – for example, paints and some cleaning materials. Moreover, the late-phase reactions may mean that symptoms emerge during the evening, several hours after you were exposed to the trigger.

But if your symptoms worsen on Monday night and do not improve until Saturday, or if Sunday and Monday are your most symptom-free days (the reaction can take time to wear off), this could point to occupational asthma. Taking regular peak flow rate measurements (see Chapter 6) can help diagnose occupational asthma.[16]

Hallmarks of occupational asthma

- Symptoms begin after starting a new job.
- Symptoms begin after a change in work conditions.
- Symptoms are better on days away from work and on holidays.

If you feel that your breathing has become impaired because of an irritant or an allergen, you may want to talk to your Health and Safety Officer and Trade Union. For legal and medical reasons your employer may ask you to undergo a number of tests to try to identify the cause of your asthma – including challenge tests (see Chapter 3). Resolving your problem may necessitate a change of environment within your company, or even, in extreme cases, looking for a new job. Compensation is available for people severely affected by occupational asthma. Contact the HSE [Health and Safety Executive] Information Services★ for a list of occupational triggers, or get in touch with the National Asthma Campaign.★

Certain professions or trades are, however, off-limits to people with asthma, owing to the high levels of allergens and/or unacceptably risky situations that such jobs would expose them to. For example, if you have asthma you should not consider becoming a welder, working with diisocyanates, flour or wood, becoming a diver or joining the armed forces.

Infective asthma

As mentioned in Chapter 2, viral infections are another common asthma trigger. Many people find that their allergic asthma deteriorates when they catch a cold, for instance. Viruses lead to a fall in lung function as well as triggering coughing and wheezing. Apart from triggering an exacerbation, some infections – such as respiratory syncytial virus (RSV) – may predispose vulnerable children to the development of allergic asthma. In other cases, viral and other lung infections can cause asthma symptoms in people without an underlying allergic condition. This is known as 'infective asthma'. The risk is especially high in some groups, such as the elderly and those with bronchitis and chronic lung conditions that cause breathlessness.

Moreover, people with long-standing (chronic) allergic asthma may be more likely to develop a respiratory tract infection than those without asthma, possibly following damage to the mucociliary escalator (see page 75). Mucus is an ideal breeding-ground for bacteria and viruses. And we've seen that people with allergic asthma may produce increased amounts of mucus that is more difficult to clear. So, if you have asthma, make sure that you are vaccinated against influenza.

Influenza

It is easy to underestimate the risks associated with influenza. To many people, flu is synonymous with a heavy cold. But influenza kills thousands of people every year. Vaccines could prevent three-quarters of these deaths, but despite this less than half the 'at risk' population (see overleaf), which includes people with asthma, are vaccinated. Influenza is dangerous to people with asthma because, like any lung infection, it can cause the condition to worsen.

The earliest definite reports of influenza date from AD 1387, while the first pandemic seems to have taken place in the sixteenth century. Pandemics have swept the world periodically ever since. Influenza mutates as it crosses the species barrier between animals and humans (and vice versa – causing, for example, outbreaks of avian influenza in Hong Kong and mainland Europe). Close contact between humans and farm animals in certain parts of the world makes it relatively easy for influenza (and, researchers increasingly realise, other infections) to jump this barrier. So any of the new strains of flu may arise in the developing world, where humans and animals still live in close proximity. Moreover, pigs are susceptible to avian and human influenza strains, and they're reared in large numbers. So pigs can act as a reservoir of infection as well as leading to the emergence of new strains to which we may not be immune.

Researchers fear that one of these strains will lead to a repeat of the Spanish Flu pandemic of 1918, which killed between 20 million and 40 million people worldwide.[17] (Between 1914 and 1918, 15 million people died directly from the first World War. So Spanish Flu possibly killed twice that number within six months.) Influenza strikes hardest at the most vulnerable people in the community – such as the elderly, people with asthma and people with heart or kidney diseases.

The government's vaccination strategy programme targets people at high risk of developing complications if they contract the flu virus. So the government recommends vaccinating all people over 65 years of age and all people in residential homes and other long-stay accommodation. It also recommends vaccinating people who are immunosuppressed (for example, those taking oral steroids or undergoing cancer chemotherapy) as well as those with the following diseases (provided that they are over six months old):

- asthma, bronchitis and chronic lung conditions that cause breathlessness
- chronic heart disease
- kidney disease
- chronic endocrine disorders, e.g. diabetes mellitus.

In other words, all allergic asthma sufferers, but especially older people and those taking oral (and probably high-dose inhaled) steroids should be vaccinated. The government does not currently recommend routine vaccination of fit children and adults. However, if asked, many GPs will vaccinate the carers of people with high-risk diseases. This means that if a carer is exposed to the virus he or she is less likely to infect the patient. If you care for someone with severe asthma you may therefore want to consider a flu jab.

The flu vaccine takes 10 to 14 days to offer protection, and immunity lasts for about six months. As influenza is rare before the middle of November, the ideal time for vaccination is October or early November; immunity then lasts throughout the winter. The vaccine's composition changes each year to reflect microbiologists' best guess at the strains likely to cause flu during the winter of that year.

However, you shouldn't be vaccinated if you are allergic to chicken or eggs – the vaccine is grown on hen's eggs. And if you have a feverish illness such as a cold you should postpone the jab until you have recovered. Side-effects associated with the jab are uncommon. Occasionally, recipients suffer soreness at the injection site. More rarely, fevers, malaise and muscle pains develop 6 to 12 hours after immunisation and can last for up to 48 hours. You should not worry that the flu vaccination can trigger influenza: the vaccine contains inactivated viruses.

Chapter summary

Asthma is a disease of the lungs that can take various forms. The most common form is allergic asthma. However, asthma can present in a variety of ways: in some cases the cause of the symptoms isn't allergic. In others, the non-allergic trigger can exacerbate or provoke allergic symptoms.

Asthma's hallmark symptoms are coughing, breathlessness and wheezing. But not everyone with asthma exhibits all the hallmark symptoms – indeed, in children and people with mild asthma, coughing may be the only symptom – and the severity of symptoms varies widely. Some people endure severe, debilitating attacks when they encounter a specific allergen.

Initially, the inflammation and symptoms characteristic of an allergic asthma attack are reversible – either spontaneously, such as when exposure to the allergen ceases, or following treatment. But prolonged inflammation can irreparably damage the lungs.

Keeping a diary of symptoms helps ensure the correct diagnosis and effective treatment. Despite the multitude of causes and forms, most people with asthma, whether allergic or non-allergic, can lead full and active lives.

Chapter 6

Asthma diagnosis and management

In this chapter we will examine the diagnosis and management of asthma. If a doctor suspects that you have asthma, he or she typically begins by taking a detailed history of your symptoms (see Chapter 5). The doctor will also aim to identify any factors that seem to exacerbate the condition. That's why keeping and summarising a diary may help (see 'An allergy diary', Chapter 3. A symptom diary for asthma works on the same principle). Your doctor might also suggest that you undergo some of the non-specific tests for allergies outlined in Chapter 3 to help assess whether you suffer from allergic asthma. (However, the fact that you are sensitive to a particular allergen doesn't necessarily mean that it is causing allergic asthma.) These tests may also help determine the allergen. But because several other diseases show similar symptoms, asthma can prove difficult to diagnose. We will look at these 'asthma mimics' first, before dealing with the specific tests for asthma.

Lung function tests show how effectively and efficiently your lungs are working. These tests help doctors diagnose asthma and determine the state of your lungs, in both allergic and non-allergic asthma. Lung function tests also help doctors determine how well the treatments are working. Symptoms aren't necessarily an infallible guide to, for example, the severity of the inflammation. And you don't want to wait until you suffer a serious exacerbation to decide that the dose of steroid, for example, needs to be higher. (Chapter 7 deals in detail with the drugs used to treat asthma.)

We'll finish by considering the treatment strategy for asthma overall and self-management plans. Self-management plans rely on using a particular lung function measurement, known as peak flow.

These plans help you take control of your asthma and allow you to tailor treatment to the severity of your symptoms. We'll conclude by looking at how you can help yourself if you suffer a severe asthma attack.

Diagnosing asthma

You might expect that doctors would find a condition as common as asthma relatively easy to diagnose – after all, they see cases almost every day. In fact, diagnosing asthma often proves difficult. As we saw in Chapter 5, there are several 'hallmark' symptoms of asthma – coughing, breathlessness and wheezing. However, symptoms vary widely from person to person and over time. Moreover, there are a number of asthma variants (see Chapter 5). Furthermore, several other diseases or conditions can mimic the symptoms. So – is your cough caused by asthma or a cold? Are you breathless at the gym because you are unfit or because you have exercise-induced asthma? Is your child wheezing because he or she has picked up a virus, or is it the first sign of asthma?

To make things more difficult, as we saw in Chapter 3 there is no definitive diagnostic test for asthma. If a doctor thinks your respiratory symptoms arise from an infection, he or she can send a sample of your phlegm to a microbiology lab to determine the bacteria responsible and assess the most appropriate antibiotic to prescribe. (Although, in practice, treatment will probably be based first on symptoms and history, resorting to microbiological testing only if the condition doesn't improve.) In contrast, none of the tests described here or in Chapter 3 can prove without any doubt that you have asthma. You may undergo a round of examinations – which, taken together, may strongly suggest that you suffer from asthma.

If you show signs of only mild asthma, your GP may make a best guess based on the history, symptoms and peak flow measurements (see pages 98–100), and then prescribe a course of anti-inflammatory drugs and bronchodilators (see Chapter 7). This 'suck-it-and-see' approach – properly called a therapeutic trial – works on the principle that if anti-inflammatory drugs and bronchodilators alleviate the symptoms and improve peak flow, you probably have asthma.

If you show little benefit, the doctor will reconsider the diagnosis. If you respond, but not as well as the doctor expects, he or she may increase the dose or refer you to a specialist – usually in respiratory medicine, but sometimes in allergies – who will perform some more advanced tests, such as challenge tests (see Chapter 3) in order to optimise treatment.

The asthma mimics

As part of confirming the diagnosis, the GP and specialist will aim to rule out the multitude of other diseases that cause symptoms similar to the hallmarks of asthma. Many diseases can mimic at least some of the symptoms of asthma – and there are too many to summarise here. But we will consider the most common.

Chronic obstructive pulmonary disease (COPD)

Chronic obstructive pulmonary disease (COPD) is one of the most important lung diseases to rule out in the diagnosis of asthma. COPD is characterised by a slow, inexorable, progressive decline in airflow. In the case of COPD, unlike that of asthma, for years healthcare professionals could do little to stem this decline – beyond persuading patients to quit smoking, which is the leading cause of COPD. Tobacco smoke is an intense irritant – which is why even passive exposure can exacerbate asthma and hay fever (see Chapter 2). But recent innovations are beginning to change the pessimistic attitude that surrounds COPD treatment.

Nevertheless, there is no doubt that quitting smoking can make a big difference to the prognosis for someone with COPD. Of all the interventions discussed in this section, stopping smoking is the most likely to lead to a marked improvement in COPD – as well as offering numerous other health benefits, not least a reduced risk of developing several cancers or heart disease.

The increasing airflow limitation, which usually occurs over several years, causes COPD's hallmark symptoms. These include awakening at night, shortness of breath, coughing and chest tightness. People with COPD are also vulnerable to infections that can lead to bronchitis (see pages 94–5), an exacerbation of their symptoms or infective asthma (see Chapter 5). Moreover, many people with COPD express high levels of inflammatory mediators (chemicals produced by the body that trigger inflammation) that 'escape' from the lungs and get into the general circulation. These mediators can produce biological changes other than lung inflammation, including weight loss and muscle wasting.[1]

Not surprisingly, COPD can dramatically undermine people's quality of life. For instance, COPD impairs job satisfaction and sex life as well as reducing the sufferer's ability to perform many of the activities of daily living that most of us take for granted.[2] In addition, COPD accounts for around 5 per cent of all deaths, killing around 30,000 people in the UK annually.

Fortunately, a growing number of drugs improve the prospects for COPD sufferers. As mentioned, giving up smoking slows the decline in lung function associated with COPD. Community pharmacists and your GP can now offer several smoking cessation measures that help determined people quit. But you still need to be committed to giving up smoking.

As COPD is very common, it is worth briefly reviewing its treatment here. In common with asthma, one type of bronchodilator (or 'reliever', which opens up the airways) – the short-acting beta$_2$-agonists (see Chapter 7) – are a mainstay of COPD therapy. But the airways of COPD patients open to a lesser extent than those in people with asthma. So short-acting beta$_2$-agonists produce less bronchodilation in people with COPD than in those with asthma. Nevertheless, short-acting beta$_2$-agonists can reduce breathlessness and improve the amount of exercise that people with COPD can take, and this makes it easier for them to perform the tasks of daily living. Short-acting inhaled beta$_2$-agonists offer effective rescue relief for attacks of breathlessness, and they could also have other benefits. For instance, these drugs might reduce the amount of bacteria that stick to cells.[3] In theory at least, this may, although it is not proven, reduce the risk of developing exacerbations.

In asthma, anticholinergic (also called antimuscarinic) bronchodilators are rarely used. In COPD, however, they dilate the bronchi more effectively than in asthma. In general, the maximum effect of ipratropium (Atrovent) and oxitropium (Oxivent) emerges after between 30 and 60 minutes and lasts for between 3 and 6 hours. Tiotropium (Spiriva) is a long-acting drug that can be used as 'maintenance therapy' (see page 106). But anticholinergic bronchodilators can cause several side-effects, such as dry mouth, nausea, constipation and headache. They can also trigger glaucoma – which is a particular problem with nebulised ipratropium. So it is important to avoid getting the drug into your eyes.

Inhaled steroids – so called 'preventers' (see Chapter 7) – may benefit people with COPD, especially, perhaps, those with severe symptoms and frequent exacerbations. Although inhaled steroids are a mainstay of allergic asthma management, their role in COPD was somewhat controversial for several years. Critics noted that any inflammation in COPD is much less marked than in allergic asthma. But in 2002 researchers published a critical examination of the evidence[4] and found that inhaled steroids reduced the number of exacerbations by 30 per cent. So inhaled steroids may be worth trying in COPD. However, if they don't make a noticeable difference after between two or three months' treatment it probably isn't worth continuing.

Doctors have used anticholinergics and short-acting beta$_2$-agonists (see Chapter 7) to treat COPD for many years. A more recent innovation combines long-acting inhaled beta$_2$-agonists and steroids. Long-acting inhaled beta$_2$-agonists are effective on their own, but the combination is more beneficial. For example, the brand Symbicort combines the steroid budesonide and the long-acting beta$_2$-agonist eformoterol (also called formoterol). In one study,[5] researchers assessed 12 months' treatment with Symbicort in people suffering from COPD. Compared to placebo (a formulation that looks the same, but does not contain either budesonide or formoterol) they found the combination improved several COPD symptoms. For example, people experienced, on average, one extra night free from awakenings a week. Symbicort also reduced the rate of mild and severe exacerbations by 62 and 24 per cent respectively compared to placebo.

Bronchitis

Chronic bronchitis – a long-lasting inflammatory disease, usually caused by smoking – is another common condition that can mimic asthma. In common with asthma, the membranes in the bronchi become inflamed and swollen. This swelling blocks the flow of air in and out of the lungs. (Indeed, some doctors consider chronic bronchitis to be a variety of COPD.) The inflammation in chronic bronchitis damages the airways and tends to trap bacteria or viruses.

In some cases, the bacteria or viruses can lead to infective asthma (see Chapter 5). In others, they lead to acute bronchitis. In the latter case, people develop the signs of a nasty 'cold' – coughing, which can be severe, phlegm, malaise, a slight fever, back and muscle pain and a sore throat. Usually, these infections are viral (so antibiotics – which work only on bacterial infections – won't do any good). Bacterial causes of acute bronchitis are less common. If you are otherwise healthy, the symptoms of acute bronchitis tend to resolve after a few days.

As mentioned, smoking usually causes the lung damage that underlies chronic bronchitis. So lung damage typical of chronic bronchitis tends to be worse than in asthma. As a result, a broncho-dilator ('reliever' – see Chapter 7) has less effect in this disease than in asthma. This degree of reversibility is one way in which doctors can differentiate chronic bronchitis from asthma. Of course, smoking-related damage to the lungs will also exacerbate asthma. The increased risk of chronic bronchitis and other lung damage is another good reason, if you need it, to quit smoking.

If you develop acute bronchitis, it's probably viral. So you should rest for a few days, make sure you drink plenty of fluids and take paracetamol, aspirin or ibuprofen (if you're not sensitive to them). If the doctor suspects that a bacteria might be the cause – for example, if you seem especially ill or your phlegm contains pus – he or she might prescribe an antibiotic. People with chronic bronchitis may receive beta$_2$-agonists (short-acting or long-acting), anticholinergics or inhaled steroids (see COPD, above, and Chapter 7).

Croup

Croup is a common childhood disease that can cause symptoms similar to asthma. Croup is caused by a virus (so don't expect antibiotics) and tends to affect the under-fives – usually during the autumn and winter. Children suffering from croup develop:

- cold-like symptoms
- a hoarse voice
- a barking cough
- wheezing on inhalation
- mild breathing problems
- mild fever (usually not above 38°C).

Croup usually improves within a week, although it may recur. While the symptoms of croup resemble those of asthma, the former tends to resolve, where as asthma tends to be persistent.

Diagnosing asthma in children

The similarity between the symptoms of croup and asthma illustrates the difficulties of diagnosing asthma in children. Some younger children, especially those under five years of age, may find the tests used for asthma – such as spirometry or using a peak flow meter (described later in this chapter) – difficult to perform. So doctors have to rely on their clinical acumen to decide whether the child suffers from asthma. Severe asthma is somewhat easier to recognise than mild asthma: symptoms so severe as to necessitate trips to the Accident and Emergency unit (A&E) are usually sufficient for a GP to diagnose severe asthma. But in many children coughing may be the main – or only – symptom of asthma. In addition, some children cough and wheeze in the night without waking their parents, who may not identify the warning signs.

If possible, keeping a diary recording the number of times that your child wakes during the night can help the doctor make a diagnosis. (A 'baby monitor' might not be much help. By amplifying every stirring, it may cause you to come rushing into the room only to find your child sleeping soundly.) You should also note whether any possible triggers – such as exercise or stroking the cat – seem to make the symptoms worse.

See page 70 for more about asthma in children.

Heart disease

Some types of heart disease mimic asthma, making diagnosis especially difficult among elderly people. For example, during a heart attack parts of the heart muscle are starved of oxygen and die. So the heart muscles weaken. As a result, the heart pumps blood less efficiently. Doctors call this condition 'heart failure'.

When the heart doesn't pump very effectively, fluid can pool in the lung – a symptom called pulmonary oedema. This pooling inhibits the transfer of oxygen across the thin lining of the alveoli.

This causes many people with pulmonary oedema to develop symptoms similar to those of nocturnal asthma (see Chapter 5), including wheezing and breathlessness. Indeed, pulmonary oedema was once known as 'cardiac asthma'. A chest X-ray usually resolves the diagnosis, and there are a growing number of treatments for heart failure that can extend life expectancy and reduce the impact of the symptoms.

It's worth remembering that asthma and heart disease are both common. So some people develop both conditions. Not surprisingly, the prospects for people with both diseases are worse than for someone with either asthma or heart disease alone.

Specific tests for asthma

As mentioned earlier, the first stage in the investigation of suspected asthma is usually to examine the history of your symptoms. Your doctor might also suggest that you undergo some of the non-specific tests for allergies outlined in Chapter 3. For example, you may be referred to a specialist for a challenge test. Here, we'll look at the two tests doctors use to assess your lung function: the peak flow meter and spirometer.

Lung function tests help diagnose asthma, assess symptom severity and monitor the response to treatment. Each test provides different and complementary information about lung function and the severity of your asthma. But your lung function measurements vary according to your sex, fitness, age and build, as well as the severity of your asthma and the effectiveness of your treatment. So, for example, peak expiratory flow rate is higher in a 20-year-old male jogger than in his 60-year-old arthritic grandmother, irrespective of any lung disease. And environmental factors, such as whether you are exposed to smoking, can influence your results from day to day.

For these reasons, lung function tests are often expressed as a percentage of the predicted average value for your sex and age group (called the per cent predicted). Your lung function will also be measured against your personal best. If you are within 85 per cent of your predicted average value, doctors regard your lung function as 'normal'. A value of 20 or even 60 per cent of your predicted value would suggest that you suffer from a lung disease.

Peak flow monitoring

Peak flow monitoring measures peak expiratory flow rate – that is, the maximum flow rate of expired air during a breath out. In other words, peak flow measures how fast you exhale. It is the most widely used lung function test. Peak flow indicates the diameter of the bronchial tubes at the time the person breathes out. This makes peak flow a very useful measure to assess the severity of lung disease and monitor response to treatment.

Peak flow meters are small enough to keep at home and are easy to use. Peak flow is most accurate when compared against your personal best. But the following figures can be used as a rule of thumb.

- Healthy people show a peak flow of 400 to 600 litres per minute. (This would be the total volume of air that your lungs could blow out in a minute if you could maintain the peak rate for 60 seconds. But don't worry: you don't have to breathe as hard as possible for an entire minute).
- People with asthma show a peak flow of 200 to 400 litres per minute.
- In severe asthma attacks, peak flow can fall to 100 litres per minute.

Often, your doctor or nurse will ask you to measure your peak flow in the morning and evening. Peak flow readings of people with asthma tend to show a greater variation over the course of the day than the measurements of those without asthma. This 'saw tooth' pattern – illustrated in Figure 6 – strongly indicates that you have asthma. In people without asthma the difference between morning and evening peak flow (called the diurnal variation) is usually less than 15 per cent. In contrast, among people with well-controlled asthma, peak flow typically varies by at least 20 per cent during the day. (In those with poorly controlled asthma the variation may be much more pronounced.) A decline in the variation in peak flow offers an indication that treatment is working.

In general, the symptoms of asthma do not usually emerge until peak flow falls by 25 per cent from your personal best. This means that measuring peak flow offers an early warning system for people with asthma. You cannot rely on symptoms alone to predict when you are likely to have an asthma attack. And by the time you begin to

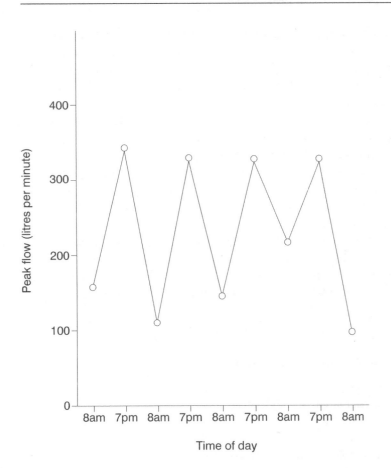

Figure 6 The 'saw tooth' peak flow pattern typical of asthma

wheeze, the inflammation is probably quite intense. Indeed, many people who develop severe asthma attacks fail to recognise worsening symptoms.

Ironically, people with severe asthma often have the worst perception of the severity of their airway obstruction. They may, for example, adapt to levels of obstruction that would provoke symptoms in someone with milder asthma – such as walking more slowly if they feel breathless. In other words, then, you need an objective measure of lung function to take steps to prevent an attack. This principle forms the basis of the self-management plans discussed later in this chapter.

So peak flow increases when your asthma is well controlled and declines when your airways narrow. For example, in people with allergic asthma, airways narrow in response to a flare-up of the underlying inflammation. Doctors aim to maintain asthma patients' peak flow to within 20 per cent of their predicted or personal best. They also try to ensure that the patients' values show minimal diurnal variation. Regular self-monitoring is, therefore, vital to ensure that your asthma is optimally controlled.

The box below summarises how to use your peak flow meter, although a doctor or nurse should instruct you and regularly ensure that you are performing the measurement correctly. Your doctor or nurse will also advise you when your peak flow meter needs replacing. In the meantime, you should wash and maintain your peak flow meter according to the manufacturer's instructions. Following these instructions and keeping your meter in a safe place where it cannot be damaged should extend its active life.

How to use a peak flow meter

- Check that the pointer is at zero.
- Sit upright or stand and lift your head.
- Hold the meter horizontally, keeping your fingers away from the pointer.
- Put the mouthpiece between your lips.
- Blow out as hard and quickly as you can.
- Take the reading, rest the pointer and begin again.
- After three readings, note the highest reading on the chart.

A word of warning, however: Don't become over-reliant on your peak flow measurement. Peak flow is not an infallible guide to symptom severity. Indeed, the level of breathlessness that different people show at any particular peak flow value varies widely. Your readings may also vary over time. So, as well as monitoring peak flow, you need to keep a note of night-time waking (see 'Nocturnal asthma' – Chapter 5) and how often you use your bronchodilator.

Spirometry

A spirometer offers another type of measurement of airway obstruction and helps confirm a diagnosis of asthma. A spirometer measures the volume of air expelled over time (see Figure 7). As you breathe out, the volume of air exhaled initially increases rapidly but then levels off to a plateau. Doctors derive three values from the spirometry curve:

- Forced expiratory volume in one second (FEV_1) – the volume of air forcefully expelled in one second.
- Forced vital capacity (FVC) – the total volume forcefully expelled when you breathe out until no further air can be expelled. (In healthy people FVC is roughly 60 per cent of the lungs' total capacity. The FVC reflects several aspects of respiration, including how 'elastic' the chest wall and lungs are and the strength of the respiratory muscles. Several diseases can reduce vital capacity, including those that lead to weakness in the respiratory muscles or chest deformity.)
- The ratio of FEV_1 to FVC.

Figure 7 shows tracings from a spirometer comparing these values for someone with asthma and someone without the condition.

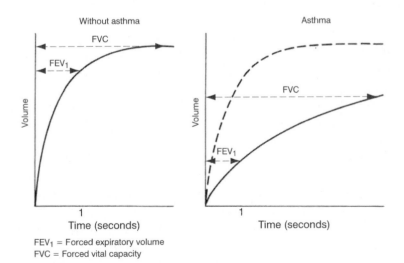

FEV_1 = Forced expiratory volume
FVC = Forced vital capacity

Figure 7 FEV_1 and FVC in people with and without asthma

101

Healthy people take about four seconds to expel a full breath. They discharge about three-quarters of their breath during the first second. In other words, they have an FEV_1:FVC ratio of 75 per cent. People with asthma have narrow airways. This means they exhale more slowly than people with normal-sized airways. So the FEV_1 declines. In most cases, FVC also declines. But the percentage decline in FEV_1 is greater than that for FVC – so the FEV_1:FVC ratio in people with asthma is, in general, lower than 75 per cent. In some cases it can be much lower.

Asthma management

In this section we'll look at self-management plans, which rely on taking regular peak flow measurements. But it is important to set these plans in the context of overall treatment. So we'll begin by considering briefly the principles of asthma management. (We'll look in detail at the drugs used to treat asthma in the next chapter.)

By the late 1980s, doctors could prescribe a number of drugs that could treat most cases of asthma effectively. So most people with asthma are able to go about their lives without their disease having a marked impact on their quality of life or their ability to perform everyday tasks. But, when these drugs were first introduced, the death rate from asthma continued to rise. So, to improve standards of care, specialists agreed a number of national and international guidelines that set the standard for asthma control and ensured that every doctor should be able to treat most of his or her patients effectively. Although there would always be some patients who fell outside the guidelines, they aimed to improve overall management.

The UK led the way with the British Thoracic Society★ Guidelines, first published in 1990. Now renamed as the British Guidelines on Asthma Management, these are regularly updated.[6] (For these reasons we won't discuss the details of the guidelines here, but will just look at the principles. Your doctor or nurse can explain the latest incarnation of the guidelines, which will take the latest research into account.)

The guidelines undoubtedly contributed to falling death rates, fewer admissions to hospital or visits to A&E, and an improved quality of life for most people with asthma in the UK. Indeed, the guidelines mean that asthmatics can now have a reasonable expectation of certain improvements from treatment, summarised in the box below. If your experience of asthma treatment does not meet these goals, it is time to consult your GP or nurse, depending who is in charge of your asthma care. (You should be reviewed regularly by a doctor or specially trained nurse in any case, probably once every three months or so.)

What to expect from asthma treatment

You can expect your treatment to:
- eliminate or minimise symptoms, during the night and day
- minimise the need for bronchodilators
- restore normal, or best possible, lung function
- reduce the risk of a severe attack or exacerbation
- minimise absence from school or work
- maintain normal activity – including exercise.

The guidelines take a 'stepped care' approach to asthma management. The central concept is a 'ladder', with five steps representing increasing asthma severity. Your symptoms and peak flow define what step you are on and, therefore, the number and dose of drugs. So if you are on the first step, for example, inhaled bronchodilators alone should suffice to control intermittent symptoms. This might be the case in some people with non-allergic symptoms, such as those with exercise-induced asthma (see page 79).

But if you need to use inhaled bronchodilators more than once a day, the doctor will probably add in an inhaled steroid or, less commonly, one of a number of other anti-inflammatories. In other words, you've moved to step two. In some cases, viral infections can trigger inflammation (see 'Infective asthma', Chapter 5). So steroids may be appropriate in some cases of infective asthma or if the infection exacerbates allergic asthma. However, most people who need steroids suffer from allergic asthma.

By the time you reach step five you'll be taking at least occasional courses of steroid tablets ('oral steroids') in addition to the inhaled medicine. Very few people suffer from asthma this severe; most will probably be at step two of the guidelines.

In essence, then, if the drugs used at one particular step fail to adequately control your symptoms, you move up the ladder. But before moving you up a step, your doctor should assess your compliance – that is, how well you are taking your drugs – and your inhaler technique. After you have spent between three and six months at any step your doctor should review your symptoms and peak flow rate. If your symptoms are well controlled you may be able to move down to a lower step.

In other words, the guidelines are dynamic. Just because you are on step two now does not mean you will stay there. Most doctors are prepared to move people up to the next step if their asthma deteriorates – but some forget the quid pro quo: moving patients back down if their asthma stabilises for a few months. When you move down a step, the dose of inhaled steroid is reduced gradually by no more than 25 to 50 per cent every three months. So if your symptoms are well controlled, discuss moving down a step with either the doctor or nurse running the asthma clinic. And don't forget that the guidelines are designed to achieve the best possible care for most people with asthma. This means that there are always exceptions, and you may be one of them – so if you feel that your asthma is poorly controlled, consult your GP or asthma nurse.

The box opposite offers some suggestions for questions to ask your doctor or asthma nurse about any treatment. You should ensure that you understand why your doctor prescribes any medicine. Asking these key questions should help you be clear about why you have been prescribed a certain drug, how to use it, and the risk of side-effects. You could ask your doctor for written instructions or to jot his or her answers down. Incidentally, most of these questions apply to any drug, not just asthma medicines.

Asking such questions allows you to take a proactive role in your asthma treatment. And, increasingly, doctors recognise the value of allowing patients to take a central place in the management of asthma and other chronic diseases. This is reflected in the growing importance of self-management plans in asthma. These plans formalise the relationship between doctor and patient, counter any misunderstanding the person with asthma might have about his or her disease, and help to alleviate poor symptom perception and feelings of helplessness.

Twelve questions to ask your doctor about your drugs

- What is the name of the drug? You should know both the brand name and the scientific or 'generic' name – e.g. Ventolin is a brand name for salbutamol. As we'll see in the next chapter, inhalers differ in their characteristics even though they contain the same generic drug. So the brand name is more important in asthma than in many other diseases.
- Is the drug an anti-inflammatory (preventer) or bronchodilator (reliever)?
- What are the side-effects?
- How likely am I to experience side-effects?
- Should I report side-effects to my doctor/pharmacist? (This applies particularly to new drugs)
- Is it a new drug? If so why is it best for me?'
- How often or in what circumstances should I take it?
- Do I need to take any precautions when I take it?
- What is the correct inhaler technique?
- Is there any risk of interactions with my other medicines, with drugs that I buy over the counter from pharmacists, or with foods or complementary therapies?
- How do I know if it is not working?
- When should I return for review?

Self-management plans

The self-management plan is built around regular peak flow readings and tailoring medication accordingly. As we've seen, taking regular peak flow readings offers an 'early warning' of an impending attack. So when your peak flow or symptoms decline to below a predetermined point – such as needing to use your bronchodilator more than once a day – you increase your dose of inhaled steroid immediately rather than waiting to see the GP. A further deterioration may trigger a course of oral steroids (which the doctor will have prescribed so that you have them to hand) or suggest an immediate visit to the GP. The final stage of the plan advises at what point you should consider going to hospital. The self-management plan works the other way, too – after your symptoms have stabilised, the plan may suggest when you can reduce your dose of steroid. If the doctor or asthma nurse is confident about your ability to follow the plan, you may be able to reduce the dose yourself. However, you should never reduce your dose without discussing the exact circumstances with your doctor or nurse. And you must always watch for any worsening of your symptoms or change in your bronchodilator use or peak flow.

Many self-management plans include graded divisions that represent peak flows. These are often known as the green, yellow and red zones. For example:

- your 'green zone' may be a peak flow of 80–100 per cent of your personal best. No change in management is required. This is your 'maintenance therapy'
- your 'yellow zone' may be a peak flow of 50–80 per cent of your personal best. You may need to double the dose of inhaled steroid until you get back to normal. You continue on this increased dose for the same number of days that it took for the peak flow to normalise. You would then return to the maintenance therapy
- your 'red zone' may be below 50 per cent of your personal best. You may need to start a week-long course of, for example, oral prednisolone or see your asthma nurse or doctor. There are certain other circumstances in which you should also arrange an appointment with your doctor (see box opposite).

Some self-management plans monitor more than peak flow readings – for example, they enable you to chart wheezing and coughing, disturbed sleep, exercise tolerance and how often you use 'rescue' bronchodilators. All of these can provide useful indicators to your condition.

Self-management plans can be extremely effective – you can monitor your lung function more frequently than any doctor. Nevertheless, the benefits of peak-flow-based self-management plans tend to be most marked among people with severe or moderate asthma – probably because this group has the biggest incentive to adhere to the plan.

When to arrange an appointment

You should arrange an appointment with your asthma nurse or doctor if you (or your child):

- wake wheezing and breathless during the night (or if your child wakes with a coughing fit)
- feel wheezy and breathless first thing in the morning
- use your bronchodilator more than usual. At most, you should use a bronchodilator once a day – any more than this suggests that your dose of anti-inflammatory drug needs increasing
- have a bad attack that is relieved only after several inhalations of bronchodilator
- develop a chest infection
- have to go to hospital because of a severe attack.

Call your emergency GP service or go to hospital if you (or your child):

- show a peak rate of less than 50 per cent of your best value
- have trouble completing a sentence within one breath
- are too breathless to eat
- are unable to stand
- become exhausted or confused.

Treating a severe asthma attack

Despite the advances in medical treatment, the guidelines for doctors and self-management plans, some people still develop severe asthma attacks. So what should you do if you or a member of your family experiences such an attack? (This advice refers to helping someone with an attack. If you are on your own, try to follow the same procedures.)

- Try to stay calm and reassure the asthmatic person.
- Ensure that they take the bronchodilator quickly and correctly.
- Ensure that they sit upright and rest their hands on your or their knees to support their back. Do not allow them to lie down, which makes it harder to breathe.
- Try to help them take slow, deep breaths – leaning on a cushion placed on their lap may help, but do not allow them to squash their stomach into their chest.

- Loosen any tight clothing.
- Get them to drink warm water – during a severe asthma attack the patient tends to breathe rapidly, which dries the mouth.
- They should take regular doses of bronchodilator. If possible, use a nebuliser or a large-volume spacer (see Chapter 7).

You should call 999 or go to Accident and Emergency if:

- the bronchodilator has not worked after five to ten minutes
- the person is clearly very distressed and unable to complete a sentence in a single breath
- the person becomes exhausted
- you are worried about their condition.

You should also call 999 if you suffer a severe attack and you are on your own.

After the attack, the doctor may prescribe a course of steroid tablets or an injection to bring the inflammation under control. If the attack necessitated an emergency call to your GP or a visit to Accident and Emergency, you should regard this as a warning that your asthma is poorly controlled. This means it is probably time to review your treatment. So following a severe attack, you should discuss several aspects of your management with your GP or asthma nurse. You should consider the following questions.

- Are you using your inhaler correctly? Poor inhaler technique reduces the amount of drug entering your lungs, undermining its effectiveness. Even if you learned correctly at the start of treatment, your technique may now be imperfect. Many people learn bad habits in using their inhaler, especially if they have not experienced severe symptoms for a while.
- Was your anti-inflammatory dose adequate? Your steroid dose will almost certainly be increased temporarily following a severe attack. You may be prescribed a short course of oral steroids after the attack. Recording peak flow allows doctors to assess how effectively your new treatment is working.
- Was there an avoidable cause? Some severe attacks occur because the person runs out of medication or because their metered dose inhaler is empty. Others are triggered by exposure to a known allergen.

- Could the symptoms have been those of an anaphylactic attack rather than severe asthma? The two are often confused (see Chapter 4).
- Did you respond correctly to the warning signs? In many cases, what appears to be a sudden attack is heralded by symptoms that last for several days but are ignored by the person with asthma (or his or her parents). Do not feel guilty about this. Rather, regard it as a hard-learned lesson.
- Does your self-management plan need updating?
- Can you do more to avoid asthma triggers? We made some suggestions for allergen avoidance in Chapter 2.

Chapter summary

Despite being common, asthma can be difficult to diagnose. There is no definite diagnostic test and several diseases can mimic asthma. But a combination of lung function tests and the general allergy tests (described in Chapter 3) help doctors determine how well the treatments are tackling the underlying inflammation. Modern drugs used in conjunction with treatment guidelines allow most people with asthma to live normal healthy lives. Many asthmatics benefit from following self-management plans. These help you take control of your asthma and allow you to tailor treatment to the severity of your symptoms. Nevertheless, if you suffer a serious asthma attack or use your bronchodilator more than once a day, it is probably time to review management.

Chapter 7

Asthma treatment

As mentioned in the last chapter, doctors treat most people with asthma by following guidelines that take a 'stepped care' approach. The central concept is a 'ladder' with five different steps, representing increasing asthma severity. Your symptoms and peak flow rate (see Chapter 6) define what step you are on and, therefore, the number and dose of drugs that the doctor prescribes. In this chapter we'll look at the drugs commonly used to treat asthma and the inhaler devices used to deliver them. Increasingly, doctors realise that separating the effects of the medicine from those of the inhaler is impossible. Each combination of 'drug plus delivery system' is unique.

This chapter can offer only a broad outline of the different drugs and inhalers available. It concentrates on the most common drugs. There are also other drugs that are used by specialists, but these are generally used only in cases of exceptionally severe, uncontrollable asthma. Several new treatments are also being assessed, including an antibody that binds to IgE[1] (we considered how this worked in Chapter 4).

You should discuss the risks and benefits of the drug and inhaler with your GP or asthma nurse, and with any drug you are prescribed you should make sure you understand its role in your asthma therapy. (See 'Twelve questions to ask your doctor about your drugs', page 105.) The range of drugs and inhalers means that your health professional should be able to find a combination that suits you and controls your symptoms.

In most cases, asthma treatment aims to deliver a 'double whammy'. A short-acting bronchodilator (also known as a 'reliever') relieves asthma attacks by opening the airways. But using a bronchodilator alone, unless the asthma is very mild, allows the underlying inflammation in the lungs (see Chapter 5, and Chapter 1 for more about the underlying immune response in allergic asthma) to rage unchecked. Using a short-acting bronchodilator alone is the medical equivalent of papering over the cracks in your home's walls caused by subsidence: you may not be able to see the cracks for a while, but the subsidence may continue unabated until your house collapses. Most people who rely solely on a bronchodilator eventually suffer a worsening of their asthma condition.

So, in addition to the bronchodilator, doctors also prescribe an anti-inflammatory (also called a 'preventer'), usually a steroid. As their name suggests, these drugs control inflammation. In other words, most people with asthma need to take a reliever occasionally to alleviate symptoms – so-called rescue medication – and also to take a preventer regularly. This dual approach to treatment, combined with regular peak flow readings and a self-management plan (see Chapter 6), dramatically reduces the likelihood of developing a serious attack.

To help you differentiate between anti-inflammatories and bronchodilators, asthma inhalers are colour-coded.

- **Anti-inflammatories** (for example, inhaled steroids) are usually brown, but may also be red, orange or yellow.
- **Bronchodilators** (for example, beta$_2$-agonists) are usually blue or green. Make sure that you understand the difference. If you are in any doubt, ask your GP or asthma nurse.

Steroids

Steroids are extremely effective at damping down the underlying inflammation that causes asthma. The production of many inflammatory mediators (see Chapter 1) is controlled by several genes. Steroids work, to a large extent, by switching off these genes – so reducing the levels of inflammatory mediators. However, this effect can take several hours to emerge, which is why steroids are ineffective as 'rescue' medication.

As the inflammation eases, the airways become less hyper-responsive (sensitive or 'twitchy' – see Chapter 5). Steroids are used in three main ways (see box overleaf) and, in inhaled form, are the mainstay of asthma therapy. Indeed, over the years, inhaled steroids have saved the lives of thousands of people with asthma and dramatically improved the quality of life of millions more.

Routes of steroid administration

- **Inhaled steroids** – including beclomethasone (also spelled beclometasone), budesonide and fluticasone – are the most common way to use steroids in asthma treatment.
- **Steroid tablets**, usually prednisolone, are used to control severe asthma.
- **Injected steroids** are used to treat acute, severe asthma attacks, usually in hospital. Injections can be used if the person is unconscious, vomiting or too distressed to swallow.

Despite their value, steroids have something of a tarnished image. Some people remain reluctant to use – or let their child take – even low-dose inhaled steroids. In part, this 'steroid phobia' reflects the problem of anabolic steroid abuse. But it's important to realise that the inhaled and oral steroids used to treat asthma are not the same as the drugs abused by some athletes, weight lifters and body builders. Anabolic steroids are chemicals related to testosterone (which is also a steroid), which increase muscle mass and, therefore, enhance physical performance. But the hazards are considerable. Anabolic steroids, such as nandrolone, can cause liver damage, depression, sexual problems and a range of other side-effects. (Despite this, anabolic steroids are occasionally used to treat serious illnesses, when the benefits outweigh the risks.)

Steroids used to treat asthma – especially protracted courses of oral steroids – can also cause side-effects. To some extent, the reluctance to use these drugs stems also from a fear of these effects. But inhaled steroids are much less likely than the tablets to cause adverse reactions. We will look in detail at the risks of these effects in the following sections on inhaled and oral steroids.

What are steroids?

In 1849, Thomas Addison told the South London Medical Society that the adrenal glands – which lie on top of the kidneys – were essential for life. But no one knew why removing the glands proved fatal. Nevertheless, Addison's disease – caused by dysfunctional adrenal glands – probably killed, among many others, Jane Austen.

In 1930, American researchers isolated a substance they called 'cortin' from the adrenal gland. Cortin injections kept animals that had their adrenal glands removed alive. It soon became clear that cortin contained several hormones – the corticosteroids. (In this chapter, unless otherwise stated, 'steroids' refers to corticosteroids.) The steroids have two main biological effects. Firstly, they regulate the metabolism of carbohydrates, such as sugar and starch, and counter inflammation. Scientists describe these as the 'glucocorticoid' effects. Secondly, steroids regulate the balance of fluid and electrolytes (minerals and salts in the blood essential for health). This affects the person's salt and water retention. These are the 'mineralocorticoid' effects.

The probability that a steroid will cause side-effects, and the type of adverse effect, depends on the balance between its mineralocorticoid and glucocorticoid effects. (We will return to this in the discussion of oral steroids, below.) Most naturally produced steroids produce both effects, to a greater or lesser extent. For example, although hydrocortisone is the main human glucocorticoid, it shows strong mineralocorticoid characteristics. Hydrocortisone cream is used to treat eczema. But, since little is absorbed through the skin, its mineralocorticoid actions don't cause serious side-effects.

Synthetic steroids developed by pharmaceutical companies separate the glucocorticoid effects from the mineralocorticoid actions. So some synthetic steroids are much stronger anti-inflammatories but are relatively weak in their effects on salt and water retention. Prednisolone, for example, is some five times more potent as an anti-inflammatory than hydrocortisone and has fairly weak mineralocorticoid action. This is, therefore, the most widely used long-term oral corticosteroid in the management of asthma and other allergic diseases.

The risk of a person developing steroid-related side-effects also depends on the dose, method of administration and duration of treatment. So, for example, the risk of developing side-effects is lower with inhaled steroids than with oral steroids. Similarly, the risk of developing side-effects is higher if you need regular doses of oral prednisolone than if you need only a course once every couple of years. As a general rule, you should take the lowest dose of steroid – inhaled or oral – that adequately controls your symptoms. This means moving down – as well as up – the five steps in the 'guidelines ladder' described in Chapter 6.

Inhaled steroids

Used regularly, inhaled steroids reduce the frequency and severity of asthma attacks. People need fewer puffs of bronchodilators (relievers) to treat acute symptoms, and lung function – measured as FEV_1 and peak flow (see Chapter 6) – usually shows a marked improvement. Indeed, the development of inhaled steroids is probably the most important advance in asthma care made so far, and these drugs are the 'gold standard' against which all new anti-inflammatories are assessed. 'Combination inhalers', which combine a steroid with a long-acting bronchodilator, are now available. See page 128.

At the time of writing, three inhaled steroids are widely used: beclomethasone (e.g. AeroBec, Becotide, Qvar), budesonide (Pulmicort) and fluticasone (Flixotide). Beclomethasone, the first inhaled steroid, was introduced in 1972, followed by budesonide and fluticasone. Fluticasone is roughly twice as potent as beclomethasone and budesonide. So the British Guidelines on Asthma Management (see Chapter 6) suggest that fluticasone be used at half the dose of budesonide or beclomethasone. This means that, at this dosage, the three steroids are equally potent. And, while there may be some subtle differences in the risk of side-effects, these seem to be marginal.

Indeed, if taken correctly, inhaled steroids cause few, if any, side-effects. One of the main concerns about the use of anti-inflammatory steroids is that they will cause 'adrenal suppression'. As we have seen, adrenal glands secrete natural steroids. The body carefully controls the amount of steroids produced by the glands, and high levels in the blood suppress the natural production. So high doses of steroids taken by people to treat inflammatory diseases (such as asthma) may suppress the production of natural corticosteroids from the adrenal glands. The greater the extent of this adrenal suppression, the more likely you are to develop some side-effects elsewhere in the body.

As a rule of thumb, doses of inhaled steroid below 800mcg beclomethasone (or its equivalent, such as 400mcg fluticasone) daily do not seem to affect adrenal function and so cause few side-effects elsewhere in the body. Some people taking long-term, high-dose inhaled steroids (1,500 to 2,000 mcg beclomethasone or equivalent daily) develop adrenal suppression to an extent that could cause side-effects more commonly associated with oral steroids (see overleaf). Fortunately, relatively few asthmatics require such high doses.

Nevertheless, there are a few side-effects linked to inhaled steroids – and you can take some steps to reduce your risk of developing these. When you use an inhaler, much of the steroid dose is either swallowed, deposited in your mouth or breathed out. The swallowed portion can be absorbed into the bloodstream in the same way as a tablet (although the dose is much lower). This distributes the steroid around the body, rather than limiting the effects to the lung. To minimise this 'systemic absorption' it is important to follow the doctor's instructions and ensure that you use your inhaler correctly. Using a spacer increases the amount of steroid reaching the lungs and decreases the amount deposited in the mouth or absorbed by the gut, and so reduces the risk of side-effects. (See later in this chapter for details of these inhaler devices).

The portion of the inhaled steroid that is deposited in the mouth can reduce oral immunity. This means that high doses of inhaled steroid can trigger an outbreak of thrush – a mild fungal disease. The yeast responsible for thrush, *Candida albicans*, causes white spots on the tongue and throat. But the oral thrush linked to inhaled steroids is rarely bad enough to require treatment. Some people taking high doses of inhaled steroid develop inflammation of the tongue (glossitis). Others develop a hoarse voice, caused when steroid deposits on the larynx (voice box). This condition, called dysphonia, is clearly a particular problem for singers, telephonists and others who use their voice for a living. Rinsing your mouth immediately after using your inhaled steroid may reduce the risk of thrush, glossitis and dysphonia. But remember to spit rather than swallow – otherwise you will increase the amount of steroid that reaches your gut.

Occasionally, high doses of inhaled steroids can cause striae – thin skin that looks like stretch marks – or lead you to bruise easily. Women are more likely to suffer from these side-effects than men, and the risk seems to increase with age. Some people can develop purpura, a rash caused when small blood vessels in the skin bleed. This is more common in older people, and isn't usually anything to worry about, but you should see your doctor if you are concerned.

High doses of inhaled steroids taken for a long time may undermine bone mass and strength. A fall in bone mass makes it more likely that a person will develop osteoporosis – brittle bone disease – which, as we'll see later, is a major problem among people taking oral steroids. People with osteoporosis are vulnerable to disabling fractures of the wrist, hip and spine.[2]

But inhaled steroids do not seem to significantly impair growth in children (a possible effect of oral steroids). Although growth velocity (the speed of the increase in height) may decline, it appears that inhaled steroids do not generally affect the final adult height.[3,4] Still, children taking inhaled steroids for a long time should have their height regularly measured by the GP or nurse running the asthma clinic.

There also seems to be a small increased risk of glaucoma and cataracts among people using inhaled steroids. Glaucoma is caused by an increase in pressure inside the eye. This damages the delicate layer of nerves – the retina – that transmits light into the brain, where it is translated into vision. Cataracts are cloudy areas in the eye's lens, which helps focus light on the retina.

While this list of side-effects may seem worrying, it's important to remember that relatively few people suffer these adverse reactions with inhaled steroids. Indeed, the marked benefits of inhaled steroids for people with asthma far outweigh the low risk of side-effects.

Oral steroids

Inhaled steroids are able to control most cases of asthma. But in some cases – if your asthma proves difficult to control or you suffer a severe worsening – your doctor may prescribe a short course of oral steroids (steroid tablets), usually prednisolone. Only a very few people with asthma need to take regular courses of oral steroids.

Oral prednisolone can be a lifesaver. Steroid tablets are usually given – for a few days in children and a week or fortnight among adults – to relieve a severe exacerbation of asthmatic symptoms. Oral steroids suppress the underlying inflammation rapidly, allowing control from day to day with inhaled steroids. But the risk of side-effects with the use of oral steroids is higher than for inhaled steroids. The likelihood of developing side-effects while taking oral steroids depends on the dose and length of treatment.

As mentioned earlier, the risk of side-effects of a steroid depends also on the balance of its glucocorticoid and mineralo-corticoid effects. The latter include raised blood pressure and changes in the body's biochemistry. Glucocorticoid adverse effects include diabetes, bone loss, stomach ulcers, muscle wasting and mental problems – such as paranoia, depression and euphoria – which, in some cases, can be severe. The box below summarises the main side-effects associated with oral steroids. High-dose oral

The possible side-effects of oral steroids

- Acne
- Cataracts
- Diabetes
- Glaucoma
- Changes in appetite
- Changes in fat distribution (typically, fat increases on the face and shoulders – known as 'moon face' and 'buffalo hump')
- Increased blood pressure
- Increased body and facial hair
- Skin thinning (steroids remove protein from the skin, causing stretch marks known as striae)
- Skin may bruise easily
- Indigestion and ulcers
- Male impotence
- Muscle weakness, especially in the limbs, shoulder and pelvis
- Fall in bone mass, leading to osteoporosis (especially in post-menopausal women) – see overleaf
- Psychological changes (including agitation, insomnia, depression and euphoria)
- Childhood growth may be retarded
- Children may become excitable

glucocorticoids can cause striae (stretch marks), acne and Cushing's syndrome – a condition characterised by changes in the shape of the face (the so-called 'moonface'), which, fortunately, often resolves after withdrawal from the drug. In children, oral corticosteroids can suppress growth. This may sound worrying, but it's important to keep the risks in perspective: uncontrolled asthma also reduces growth and might adversely affect adult height.

Bone loss

Bone loss induced by long-term oral steroids poses a particular problem as the proportion of older people in the population increases. Bone mass declines because the skeleton – despite appearances – is not inert. The stresses and strains of daily life lead to micro-fractures – tiny cracks in the bones. Left unresolved, these micro-fractures would undermine the skeleton's strength, so old bone is replaced with new bone throughout life. Depending on its location in the body, between 3 and 25 per cent of the bone is replaced each year.

During this 'remodelling', a group of cells known as osteoclasts break down old bone by forming microscopic pits on the bone's surface. Another group of cells – the osteoblasts – fill these pits with new bone. So the body needs a continual supply of raw material – calcium and vitamin D. Most of the vitamin D is formed by sunlight on the skin and from our diet. But not everyone gets enough vitamin D. Vegans, older people and some Asian or Afro-Caribbean women (if their skin is covered up in sunlight) are especially at risk of vitamin D deficiency. To ensure you get enough of both minerals, you should take 10 to 20 mcg of vitamin D and 1,000 to 1,500 mg of calcium daily to prevent osteoporosis. This means drinking roughly a litre (two pints) of milk a day. This is true for everyone, but it is especially important to take sufficient vitamin D and calcium if you're taking steroids.

Oral steroids throw the delicate balance of bone remodelling into disarray. During long-term use they reduce bone formation by up to 25 per cent, through three linked actions:

- steroids inhibit the production of new bone
- people taking oral steroids excrete more calcium in their urine than non-users
- people taking oral steroids absorb less calcium from food than non-users.

This combination of increased calcium excretion and reduced absorption means that less calcium is available to build new bone. As a result, people taking long-term oral steroids are much more likely to suffer a fracture – post-menopausal women are especially vulnerable because the steroids' actions add to the normal age-related decline in bone mass.

The effect of oral steroids on the skeleton is most marked during the first six months of treatment, when people can lose between 5 and 15 per cent of their bone mass. After this, the loss slows to about 2 per cent annually, but increases with higher doses and longer duration of treatment. As a rule of thumb, bone loss becomes clinically significant when the dose reaches 7.5 mg a day of prednisolone or the equivalent dose of other glucocorticoids, or treatment lasts for more than three months.[2] So if you are taking oral steroids, you should:

- discuss taking anti-osteoporosis drugs – such as a group of drugs known as the bisphosphonates or calcitriol (Rocaltrol) – with your doctor
- ask your doctor to refer you for a bone scan to determine the extent of any bone loss
- make sure that you follow a bone-healthy lifestyle (see box).

Lifestyle strategies to prevent bone loss

- Take weight-bearing exercise (such as rapid walking, jogging and aerobics) for at least 20 minutes, three times a week.
- Avoid smoking.
- Avoid excessive alcohol consumption.
- Hormone replacement therapy (HRT) for post-menopausal women can stem the decline in bone mass. However, it is associated with several side-effects. You should discuss the risks and benefits fully with your doctor.
- Ensure your calcium and vitamin D intakes are adequate – this may mean taking supplements.

Other adverse effects
Steroids may be associated with a number of other potentially serious problems. As we saw earlier when discussing inhaled steroids,

steroids can cause 'adrenal suppression'. Hormones produced by the adrenal glands help you cope with the stress of infections and injury, including surgery – and oral steroids can blunt this response. So people who contract an infection, are injured or who require surgery might need an increased steroid dose to compensate for the reduced production of natural hormones. Furthermore, people who stopped treatment with more than 10 mg prednisolone or equivalent within three months before the accident or operation might need to re-start treatment. For this reason, people on long-term oral steroids should carry a steroid treatment card to alert health professionals to the drug dose and duration. You should also tell any doctor, dentist, nurse or midwife that you are taking, or have taken, oral steroids. You could consider wearing a MedicAlert bracelet or a similar device that gives the dose and type of steroid in case you become unconscious. This alerts doctors and other healthcare professionals to the fact that you have a medical condition. Contact the MedicAlert Foundation★ for more information.

Chronic (long-term) oral corticosteroids can also increase the risk of contracting an infection, exacerbate its severity and lead to unusual symptoms. Indeed, doctors may recognise some diseases – such as septicaemia or tuberculosis – only at a relatively advanced stage among people taking oral corticosteroids. People without immunity to chickenpox or measles may need immunisation. If you think you or your child is beginning to develop chicken pox or measles during, or within several months after, a course of oral steroids, consult your GP. The following are signs to watch for.

- Some children and most adults may feel ill and experience a fever, headache or cough before the chickenpox rash erupts. Measles may be preceded by a fever, a hacking cough and red eyes (conjunctivitis).
- Chickenpox is heralded by a crop of raised spots, which develop pus-filled heads and may burst, crust or disappear. This stage lasts for about five days and may be accompanied by a fever. Spots tend to appear on the trunk rather than on the limbs.
- Measles is characterised by Koplik's spots: these look like small, white grains of sand surrounded by inflammation. They tend to develop on the gums. The skin rash begins in front of and

below the ears as well as on the neck. Spots spread rapidly to the trunk and arms as they fade on the face.

You should also consult your GP if you develop diarrhoea, a fever or vomiting while taking oral steroids.

Withdrawal from oral steroids

If you've been on oral steroids for a while, your doctor may decide that you should not stop them suddenly. In some people, rapidly withdrawing oral steroids can impair production of natural steroids by the adrenal glands, induce dangerously low blood pressure and, in a few cases, even lead to death. Moreover, rapid withdrawal can cause several other symptoms, including fever, muscle and joint pains, rhinitis, conjunctivitis and weight loss.

So if your asthma is unlikely to relapse and you fall into one of the groups in the box below, your doctor may decide to withdraw the oral corticosteroids gradually. You should never simply stop taking any drug, especially oral steroids, without talking to your doctor first, however well you feel.

When to withdraw oral corticosteroids slowly

You should not stop oral steroids suddenly if you:

- are taking a repeat course (especially for longer than three weeks)
- are taking a short course within a year of stopping long-term treatment
- have other causes of adrenal suppression
- are taking more than 40mg prednisolone daily (or equivalent)
- take repeat doses in the evening
- have been on more than three weeks' treatment.

Weighing up the risks and benefits

The risk of side-effects means that, as a general rule, you should take the lowest dose of oral corticosteroid for the shortest time that adequately controls your symptoms. You should regularly review the risks and benefits of continuing oral steroids with your doctor or asthma nurse. And consult your doctor if you think you are suffering unacceptable side-effects. Nevertheless, it's important to remember that oral steroids alleviate the disability arising from asthma and other allergic diseases. And they save the lives of countless people. Despite their limitations, oral steroids are invaluable.

Other anti-inflammatories

A number of other drugs can also alleviate inflammation by acting in a different way from steroids. These avoid steroid-related side-effects. However, they tend not to be as effective as steroids. For this reason, inhaled steroids remain the mainstay of asthma treatment.

Sodium cromoglycate

Sodium cromoglycate (also spelled cromoglicate and available as brands including Cromogen, Intal), introduced into conventional medicine in 1967, was isolated from the seeds of a Middle Eastern plant, *Ammi visnaga*, which is related to the carrot and was used to treat asthma by traditional healers for centuries.

When inhaled, sodium cromoglycate 'stabilises' mast cells, preventing them from degranulating and releasing their cocktail of inflammatory mediators (see Chapter 1) that can contribute to allergic asthma and to some non-allergic forms, such as exercise-induced asthma. This targeted action means that sodium cromoglycate is a less effective anti-inflammatory than inhaled steroids (mast cells, as we saw in Chapter 1, aren't the only source of the mediators that lead to asthma). So if you or your child does not respond well within four to six weeks, you should consider switching to inhaled steroids. Side-effects caused by sodium cromoglycate can include rash, headache and upset stomach, especially among young children with mild asthma, but these are rare. The drug is now rarely used, even in children. Large analyses of clinical trials have concluded that sodium cromoglycate offers little long-term benefit.[5]

Nedocromil sodium

Nedocromil sodium (Tilade) has been used as an inhaled preventer in people with mild asthma. However, nedocromil is less effective than inhaled steroids and so is now rarely prescribed.

In addition to 'stabilising' mast cells, nedocromil also reduces the irritation of nerves in the lung and, as a result, may sometimes be effective against coughing. It is useful in preventing exercise-induced asthma, particularly when taken 20 minutes before working out. Nedocromil is also especially effective in children, but they must be over six years of age (the drug has not been formally approved for younger children).

Inhaled nedocromil is not, however, as potent as the inhaled steroids. So if your or your child's symptoms do not improve after six to eight weeks your doctor might switch you to inhaled steroids. Side-effects of nedocromil are relatively uncommon, but include headache, nausea, vomiting and indigestion. Nedocromil comes in a 'mint' flavour that aims to hide the unpleasant taste that inhaling the drug can leave in your mouth.

Leukotriene receptor antagonists

In 1938, scientists injected cobra venom into the lung of a guinea pig, causing bronchoconstriction. At that time, researchers believed that histamine caused the bronchoconstriction characteristic of asthma. But antihistamines did not alleviate the venom's effect on the guinea pig. This suggested that some other substance was responsible. Later studies showed that other chemicals triggered the release of this same 'mystery mediator'. And in 1979 researchers finally discovered that the substance was a cocktail of three inflammatory mediators called leukotrienes. These mediators – released by mast cells (see Chapter 1) – potently constrict the bronchi and stimulate mucus secretion.

These discoveries led to the development of montelukast (Singulair) and zafirlukast (Accolate), members of the first new class of anti-inflammatory for asthma to be launched in 20 years. Montelukast and zafirlukast – unlike inhaled steroids, nedocromil and cromoglycate – are tablets rather than given by inhalers. They reduce the likelihood of bronchoconstriction following allergen exposure, exercise, irritants and aspirin (see Chapter 5). These 'leukotriene receptor antagonists' work in a similar way to antihistamines – by binding to specific receptors on the surface of cells that, when stimulated, generate inflammatory symptoms. They 'sit' in the leukotriene receptor, preventing the leukotrienes from binding and activating the cell's 'machinery'.

Side-effects linked to leukotriene receptor antagonists, which include headache and gastrointestinal disturbances, tend to be mild. Despite this, leukotriene receptor antagonists used alone are not recommended for most people because they are considerably less effective than low-dose inhaled steroids. They have been used as an 'add-on' treatment to inhaled steroids, but are much less effective in combination than long-acting bronchodilators (see below).[6,7]

Other research, however, suggests that adding montelukast to fluticasone controls asthmatic symptoms to a similar degree as adding salmeterol to the inhaled steroid (see 'Combination inhalers', page 128). In one study,[8] two groups of asthma patients were inadequately controlled on fluticasone alone. After adding either montelukast or salmeterol, in both groups far fewer suffered an asthma exacerbation than would normally be expected if their condition remained poorly controlled.

Bronchodilators

Bronchodilators – also called relievers – are almost always used in conjunction with anti-inflammatories (preventers). There are two types of bronchodilator; short-acting and long-acting. The short-acting bronchodilators rapidly alleviate acute asthma symptoms. So even if you don't use them very often, it is essential to keep a spare short-acting bronchodilator to hand as 'rescue' treatment in case you suffer an unexpected asthma attack. The long-acting bronchodilators do not act quickly enough to alleviate acute asthma.

Ideally, you should keep the extra inhaler of short-acting bronchodilator with you at all times, or at least where it will be accessible – although if you have been taking your drugs correctly, monitoring your peak flow and following a self-management plan, an attack out of the blue should be rare.

As we saw earlier, bronchodilators do not reduce the underlying inflammation in the lungs that is responsible for most asthma symptoms. So it is important to continue taking your anti-inflammatory, even when you feel well, and even if you are taking a long-acting bronchodilator.

Short-acting beta$_2$-agonists

The most widely used bronchodilators, a group of drugs known as 'short-acting beta$_2$-agonists', have been used for more than 30 years to manage asthma.

As we have seen, many drugs work by either blocking or stimulating receptors on various cells in the body, for example, on nerves and muscles. The beta$_2$-receptor helps control lung muscles. These receptors normally respond to adrenaline, a stress hormone that makes our bodies ready to fight or escape, and noradrenaline, a chemical that carries messages from nerves to muscles (a so-called neurotransmitter).

Adrenaline and noradrenaline relax muscle surrounding the airways and clear mucus by encouraging cilia to beat more rapidly (see Chapter 5 for more about the lungs' natural defence system). The short-acting beta$_2$-agonists bind to and stimulate beta$_2$-receptors, mimicking the action of adrenaline and noradrenaline.

To illustrate this, imagine that the beta$_2$-receptor is the ignition lock on a car. The cell is the car. And adrenaline and noradrenaline are both keys. When either key fits into the lock, the car starts. That is, the nerve or muscle cell's 'internal machines' start and you get the response. Now imagine that you have another key that fits into the ignition – the beta$_2$-agonist. It's like a master passkey. It sits in the receptor and activates the cell's internal machinery. So beta$_2$-agonists open the airways, for between three and six hours.

Salbutamol (e.g. Airomir, Aerolin, Ventolin) and terbutaline (Bricanyl) are the most widely prescribed short-acting beta$_2$-agonists. Usually, beta$_2$-agonists are inhaled, although a sustained-release tablet containing salbutamol is available. The inhalers take four to ten minutes to work. The tablet takes longer, though bronchodilation tends to be more sustained than with the inhalers. However, the likelihood of developing side-effects is higher than with the inhalers, which means that sustained-release salbutamol is not widely used. Syrups containing beta$_2$-agonists, which can help some children with occasional symptoms, are available – although generally inhalers are less likely to cause side-effects. There are also injectable beta$_2$-agonists, which may be used in hospital to treat severe attacks. Beta$_2$-agonists can also be used in a nebuliser (see pages 138–9).

In general, inhaled short-acting beta$_2$-agonists are safe. However, at high doses they can bind to another type of beta-receptor – the beta$_1$-receptor – in heart muscles. These help control heart function. The binding of beta$_2$-agonists stimulates the heart, so people may develop cardiovascular side-effects, including palpitations, tremor and arrhythmia (abnormal heartbeat).

Furthermore, using short-acting beta$_2$-agonists regularly can mean that the receptors respond less well over time – a problem known as tolerance or tachyphylaxis. When this happens, you need to take increasing amounts of the drug to get the same effect. Short-acting beta$_2$-agonists may cause you to develop tolerance in two ways. Firstly, the body 'adapts' to the high levels of the drug by 'switching off' some beta$_2$-receptors. Secondly, short-acting beta$_2$-agonists reduce the amount of natural anti-inflammatory steroids produced by the body. For these reasons, regular use of short-acting beta$_2$-agonists does not offer real benefits and will not improve either your symptoms or quality of life. You should, therefore, use these drugs only to alleviate an acute attack. You should use one of the preventers, usually an inhaled steroid, to control the underlying inflammation.

Long-acting bronchodilators

While short-acting beta$_2$-agonists keep the bronchi open for between three and six hours, another group of drugs – long-acting bronchodilators – keep the airways open for up to 24 hours when used twice daily. Unlike the short-acting beta$_2$-agonists, you use these regularly, and they are not effective as 'rescue medication'. And, like the short-acting bronchodilators, they have little if any effect on inflammation. So long-acting bronchodilators must always be used with an anti-inflammatory (preventer). However, long-acting bronchodilators can dramatically improve lung function, so may mean the dose of steroid does not need to be increased. There are currently two long-acting inhaled bronchodilators on the market, salmeterol and eformoterol (sometimes spelled formoterol), as well as two tablets, bambuterol and sustained-release theophylline.

Salmeterol

Salmeterol (Serevent) is a beta$_2$-agonist with a long duration of action. Beta$_2$-agonists are 'reversible' drugs – they bind to the receptor then dissociate and bind to another receptor. But salmeterol has a long 'tail'. The 'active' end – the part that produces the therapeutic effect – binds to a specifc region on the beta$_2$-receptor: the active site. The other end of the chain anchors itself very strongly to another part of the beta$_2$-receptor. This means the active end of the salmeterol remains in close proximity to the active site on the receptor. So it 'bounces' in and out of contact with the receptor's active site – like a spring – activating it repeatedly. As a result the bronchi remain open for 12 hours after a single dose. To ensure 24-hour effectiveness you take salmeterol twice daily (morning and evening). The long duration of action means that salmeterol is especially effective against nocturnal asthma.

The side-effects of salmeterol are those common to other beta$_2$-agonists, such as tremor, increased heart rate and palpitations. These effects are usually minor and decline during regular use. But you should not use salmeterol to alleviate an acute attack – use short-acting inhaled beta$_2$-agonists instead. Salmeterol can take 20 minutes to exert its maximum effect, so it is relatively ineffective in an acute asthma attack. So, again, always carry your short-acting bronchodilator in case you need to use 'rescue' medication.

Eformoterol

Eformoterol (Foradil, Oxis) is also a beta$_2$-agonist with a long duration of action, but works in a different way from salmeterol. Rather than 'bouncing' in and out of contact with the beta$_2$-receptor's active site, eformoterol binds strongly to the active site and is absorbed by the fatty membrane surrounding each cell. When eformoterol levels in the blood fall, the drug slowly leaches out of the fat. This results in a long duration of action. The side-effects and effectiveness of eformoterol – for example, improvements in lung function, nocturnal symptoms and reduced use of 'rescue' bronchodilators – appear to be similar to those produced by salmeterol. Eformoterol acts more rapidly than salmeterol. Nevertheless, it is still not appropriate as a 'rescue' bronchodilator.

Combination inhalers

Combination inhalers that include a fixed dose of long-acting $beta_2$-agonist and a steroid have now been introduced. At the time of writing, two combination inhalers are on the market: Seretide, which contains salmeterol and fluticasone, and Symbicort, which contains eformoterol and budesonide. (Symbicort is also valuable in the treatment of COPD – see Chapter 5).

Combination inhalers are very useful for most people with chronic asthma. Many find using a single inhaler instead of two separate inhalers more convenient. They also find it is easier to remember to take the inhaler regularly, as they get an immediate relief of symptoms from the bronchodilator. For example, a study from Sweden[9] compared six months' treatment with Symbicort against budesonide and eformoterol delivered using separate inhalers in 321 adults with asthma. Nine per cent of Symbicort users stopped treatment, compared with 19 per cent of those using the two inhalers, which seems to indicate that people were more likely to stick to treatment with Symbicort.

Other studies[10] show that asthma can be controlled with lower doses of inhaled steroid by using combination inhalers. American researchers combined the results of four studies assessing fluticasone and salmeterol delivered from combined or separate inhalers. Taken together, the studies showed that using a single inhaler improved morning peak flow (see pages 98–100) compared with using separate inhalers. Indeed, people using a single inhaler were around 40 per cent more likely to show an increase of either 15 or 30 litres per minute, which doctors regard as good responses to treatment.

Bambuterol

Bambuterol (Bambec) is a tablet that is broken down by the body to release an active ingredient: the $beta_2$-agonist terbutaline. The slow release from the tablet produces a sustained effect. As mentioned above, oral $beta_2$-agonists are more likely than the inhaled variety to provoke side-effects, including tremor and headache. Bambuterol is not approved for children and you shouldn't take it during pregnancy.

Theophylline

Theophylline is a member of a family of chemicals – the xanthines – which includes caffeine and theobromine. Indeed, you probably drink theophylline every day: tea contains small amounts. Xanthines relax the ring of muscle surrounding the bronchi. Theophylline also loosens the bronchial mucus, so unblocking the airways.

Theophylline (e.g. Nuelin, Slo-Phyllin, Uniphyllin) is given as a sustained-release tablet, meaning that the active ingredient is slowly released into the gut. This keeps the bronchi open for up to 12 hours. Unlike the other long-acting bronchodilators, theophylline acts partly by blocking an enzyme called phosphodiesterase (PDE), which controls the duration of messages inside the cell. (So it's different from the beta$_2$-agonists, which act on receptors on the outside of the cell.) Different cells produce different types of PDE. Many of the cells involved in inflammation in asthma produce a subtype of this enzyme, called PDE4. Several drugs that block PDE4 – the PDE4 inhibitors – are now being developed as new treatments for asthma and COPD.

Theophylline has been used as a bronchodilator since 1922. (A related drug, aminophylline – Phyllocontin Continus – is similar in action and side-effects to theophylline.) But for many years it was a drug on the wane. This was largely because, at blood levels relatively close to those that open the airways, theophylline tends to cause a number of unpleasant side-effects – similar to those you might feel if you drink too much caffeine: abdominal pain, diarrhoea, headache, heart disturbances, insomnia, nausea, nervousness, tremor and vomiting. The risk of side-effects means that the dose must be carefully tailored to the person's response. You take increasing amounts of theophylline until either the asthma is controlled or side-effects emerge. And, to ensure levels remain within safe limits, people taking theophylline may need regular blood tests.

Furthermore, many external factors influence the way the body metabolises (breaks down) theophylline, which can make it ineffective or produce unacceptable side-effects. Smoking and heavy alcohol use, for example, lower blood levels of the drug, which may make it ineffective as a bronchodilator. Similarly, viral infections, heart failure and liver disease can raise blood levels – sometimes into the toxic range – and a wide range of other drugs (see box overleaf for some examples) can also affect theophylline levels in the blood.

Because of this, you should check with your doctor or pharmacist about drug interactions. You must mention that you take theophylline if you are prescribed a new drug or ask for over-the-counter medication.

Examples of drugs that can interact with theophylline

- Some antibacterials – such as ciprofloxacin (Ciproxin), clarithromycin (Klaricid) and erythromycin (e.g. Erymax, Erythroped, Erythrocin)
- Some antidepressants – including fluvoxamine (Faverin) and St John's Wort
- Fluconazole (Diflucan) and ketoconazole (Nizoral) – antifungals
- Calcuim channel blockers (for high blood pressure and angina), such as diltiazem (e.g. Tildiem, Adizem, Dilcardia) and verapamil (Cordilox, Securon, Univer)
- Cimetidine (e.g. Dyspamet, Tagamet) – an ulcer-healing drug

---

However, as well as being a bronchodilator, theophylline is also an anti-inflammatory – it seems to inhibit T-lymphocytes, a type of white blood cell involved in allergic asthma (see Chapter 1). And, importantly, the anti-inflammatory effects emerge at doses below those that cause bronchodilation – so anti-inflammatory doses are below those that may lead to side-effects. Although theophylline is not a particularly powerful anti-inflammatory, this effect is one reason the PDE4 inhibitors could be a promising future treatment for asthma. Researchers also hope that the newer drugs will cause fewer side-effects.

In the meantime, theophylline is used more as an anti-inflammatory in combination with inhaled steroids. It is effective in people who have severe asthma, where it has been shown to be a useful 'add-on therapy'. Now that lower doses than previously are used, side-effects are not such a problem.

Anticholinergics

Anticholinergics are usually prescribed when high-dose inhaled steroids combined with salmeterol (see 'Combination inhalers', page 128) fail to control a person's symptoms adequately. Two inhaled anticholinergics – ipratropium bromide (Atrovent) and oxitropium bromide (Oxivent) – are currently available for asthma, although they are rarely used. However, they may be useful in older people, and may be particularly effective in COPD (see Chapter 5).

We know that many drugs work by either blocking or stimulating receptors on cells. The 'cholinergic' receptors in the bronchi respond to a neurotransmitter (a chemical that carries messages from nerves to muscles) called acetylcholine. When this binds to the receptors the bronchi contract. Anticholinergics block the cholinergic receptors, preventing acetylcholine from binding, so keeping the airways open. The full effects of ipratropium and oxitroprium tend to emerge relatively slowly, but altogether the former keeps the bronchi open for up to eight hours and the latter for about twelve hours.

Side-effects are rare. But people with glaucoma (an increase in the pressure inside the eye, which can damage the retina) and benign prostatic hyperplasia (see below) should use anticholinergics with caution, especially if taken via a nebuliser (see pages 138–9). If you are taking nebulised anticholinergics, be sure to use a mouthpiece. Some people with glaucoma, especially those who do not use nebulisers with a mouthpiece, may find anticholinergics increase the pressure in the eye, thereby speeding the destruction of the retina. Benign prostatic hyperplasia is a non-cancerous enlargement of the prostate gland (which lies, in men, at the base of the bladder surrounding the urethra – the tube urine passes through). This enlargement causes a variety of urinary symptoms, including incontinence. In men with this condition, anticholinergics can trigger a worsening of symptoms and hinder the ability to pass urine.

Inhaler devices

We have seen that a wide range of preventers and relievers are available to treat asthma. But the safety and effectiveness of the drugs themselves are not the end of the story. To be most effective, the medicine needs to reach the lungs. This is not a problem with oral drugs, which are transported to the lungs by the blood. Most asthma drugs, however, are inhaled to reduce the risk of side-effects. Your choice of inhaler device can strongly influence the effectiveness of treatment and the risk that you will develop side-effects. Inhaler devices fall into three main groups:

- metered-dose inhalers
- dry-powder inhalers
- breath-actuated devices.

In addition, spacers are devices that can be used with metered-dose inhalers to improve their effectiveness. Nebulisers can be used by people with severe asthma or those who are unable to use inhaler devices.

There are a large number of different inhalers available and, while the choice appears confusing, at least this means you can work with your doctor or nurse to individualise treatment. If you find one inhaler difficult to use, ask your doctor or nurse to prescribe an alternative.

Metered-dose inhalers

Pressured metered dose inhalers (MDIs) – for example, Airomir and Evohaler – are used to deliver bronchodilators and inhaled sterods. MDIs, which are sometimes known as 'puffers', are the most common way to deliver drugs for asthma. However, there are two main problems with MDIs. Firstly, although people usually shake the inhaler to see if they are running out of medication, MDIs contain enough propellant (the gas that carries the active drug and makes the sound) for about 30 more actuations (pressing actions) than the number of doses of drug in the inhaler. As a result, it is possible to inhale nothing but propellant when you reach the end of a canister – you cannot tell from the sound that the propellant no longer contains the drug. Obviously, if this is the case, there is a greater risk that you will suffer an asthma attack.

The second problem is that many people use MDIs incorrectly. The aerosol spray containing the drug exits the inhaler at 15 metres per second – that's 75 miles per hour. This means that once you press the inhaler, you have just 0.1 or 0.2 seconds to inhale. Not surprisingly, timing faults are the most common error in inhaler technique among people using MDIs. Poor timing means that less drug reaches the lungs and more is deposited in the mouth and throat. This increases the risk of side-effects from inhaled steroids (see pages 114–116) and reduces the effectiveness of both anti-inflammatories and bronchodilators.

A number of other common technique faults reduce the amount of drug reaching the lung:

- stopping inhaling when the cold jet of propellant hits the back of the throat (doctors describe this as the 'cold Freon' effect)
- actuating (pressing) the inhaler too early or too late – before or after breathing in
- pressing the canister twice during the same breath
- not placing the mouthpiece correctly in the mouth
- puffing out the cheeks (which traps the drug in the corners of the mouth).

So, how can you use an MDI correctly?

- Remove the mouthpiece cover and check that the mouthpiece is clean and clear of any obstruction. If you leave an inhaler in your pocket without the cover, fluff and even coins can become caught in the mouthpiece.
- Shake the inhaler well. In many cases, particles of drug 'float' on the propellant. Shaking the MDI ensures that each actuation delivers an equal amount of the drug.
- Cold canisters can reduce the amount of drug delivered from an MDI. So on cold days warm the inhaler in your hands. However, do not dismantle the MDI or place it on a heater or radiator.
- Breathe out as far as you can and place your lips around the mouthpiece. Leaving your mouth open can lead to the drug being deposited on the lips, face and teeth.
- Breathe in steadily and press – 'actuate' – the device. Breathing in slowly and steadily reduces turbulence in the upper airways, so more drug reaches the lower airways.
- Hold your breath for ten seconds, if possible. Holding your breath increases the amount of small particles deposited on the airway walls.
- If you need more than one puff, wait a minute before beginning again. Always shake the canister between doses.
- Replace the mouthpiece cover.

Many older people, particularly those with arthritis or rheumatism, do not have the hand strength to operate an MDI – actuating an inhaler requires about 6lbs of pressure. You could try actuating a standard MDI using two hands, or use a dry-powder inhaler (see opposite) that will not require any pressure. If someone is available to help you, he or she could actuate your MDI as you inhale the medication through a spacer (see opposite). Another option is to use a 'Haleraid', which provides an add-on arm to your inhaler, allowing you to work a metered-dose inhaler with the palm of your hand. It fits most, but not all, metered-dose inhalers. The Haleraid also allows a metered-dose inhaler to be fitted to a spacer (though not snugly) – the drawback is that you still have to co-ordinate actuation and inhalation. Your doctor, nurse or pharmacist can advise you which inhalers the Haleraid fits. The Arthritis Research Campaign* offers further advice and support for people living with this debilitating condition.

At present, some MDIs are propelled with chlorofluorocarbons (CFCs). Although CFCs are harmless to the lungs, when released into the atmosphere they damage the ozone layer. This 'hole' in the ozone layer allows more harmful ultra-violet (UV) light to penetrate to earth. For this reason CFCs are being phased out and it is likely that those used as propellants in MDIs will be withdrawn altogether over the next few years.

The new non-CFC propellants used in MDIs have undergone extensive safety tests. Indeed, the testing was more extensive than that originally carried out on CFC propellants. CFC-free inhalers are safe, but you may experience some changes if switching to the new version. The 'flavour' of the new propellant, as well as the sensation of the propellant in the mouth, may differ from the old inhalers. The inhaler may also be a different shape, feel and weight. Nevertheless, most people consider the inhalers containing the new propellant to be just as acceptable as the CFC versions. Changing to environmentally friendly inhalers may affect your drug dose.

Changing a tried-and-trusted inhaler is always stressful, but it is important to remember that the new versions are as effective and safe as your existing medicine. Nevertheless, it is prudent to monitor your symptoms and peak flow during the switch. Remember too that the CFC-free inhalers can vary in their characteristics and should be prescribed by brand.

Dry-powder inhalers and breath-actuated devices

Dry-powder inhalers (DPIs) – for example, Accuhaler, Diskhaler, Clickhaler, Turbohaler – and breath-actuated devices, such as the Autohaler, are triggered when you inhale and are available containing a variety of bronchodilators and anti-inflammatories. Unlike MDIs, you do not have to actuate the inhaler, which reduces the need for co-ordination and manual dexterity. There are differences between the various inhalers, so make sure you understand how to use yours and ask for the information leaflet provided by the manufacturer.

DPIs and breath-actuated devices increase the amount of drug deposited in the lung. Indeed, steroid doses delivered by the Turbohaler are only half that delivered from an MDI. DPIs and breath-actuated devices generally produce a greater increase in peak flow, and people may need fewer doses of 'rescue' medication compared with MDIs. Nevertheless, DPIs and breath-actuated devices still need a certain amount of manual dexterity to be used correctly. And individual devices have advantages and disadvantages – so make sure that you discuss these with your doctor or nurse. One disadvantage of DPIs and breath-actuated inhalers is that they cannot be used with a spacer (see below). In addition, the speed at which you inhale influences the amount of drug deposited in the lungs.

Overall, the advantages of DPIs and breath-actuated inhalers seem clear. However, while cost-containment in the National Health Service remains of overriding importance, MDIs offer one critical advantage: they are cheap – which is one reason why they remain widely prescribed. If you are not happy with your inhaler, ask your doctor or nurse about switching to a different one.

Spacers

Spacers are used with MDIs. There are various types, but all reduce the amount of drug deposited in the mouth, increase the proportion reaching the lungs and overcome the 'cold Freon' effect mentioned earlier. As less steroid remains in the mouth and more reaches the lungs, the risk of local side-effects, such as thrush, is less than with MDIs used alone. And less drug in the mouth means there is less to swallow, so the risk of other side-effects may also be reduced. If you use an MDI, steroid doses of above 800mcg of beclomethasone or budesonide, or 400mcg of fluticasone, should be administered using a large-volume spacer.

Inhalers and spacers come in various shapes and sizes. Manufacturers make spacers to fit their own brand of MDI, so you need to use the correct inhaler and spacer. Some MDIs now have an integral spacer – these are easier to use than a separate spacer and traditional MDI. See the box opposite for information on using a spacer correctly.

Large-volume spacers, also called chamber devices, come in two clear plastic sections that you clip together. A valve at one end of the spacer opens only when you breathe in and shuts when you breathe out. In this way, large-volume spacers hold the drug particles in suspension until you inhale them. This means there is no need to co-ordinate actuation and inhalation. However, large-volume spacers are unwieldy and do not fit easily into a bag or pocket. This makes taking asthma drugs more obvious, especially in social situations. Teenagers, especially, may feel that the large-volume spacer draws attention to their asthma.

Tube spacers – the simplest type of spacer – aim to strike a balance between portability and the benefits of the larger spacers. A short tube is attached to the end of the inhaler, which allows the propellant to evaporate. This reduces the 'cold Freon' effect and slows the particles, which increases the amount of drug that reaches the lung. However, some co-ordination is still needed to use the device and tube spacers are unsuitable for children under five. The AeroChamber is a small and compact tube spacer. It contains a valve that 'whistles' if you inhale too quickly.

Before the age of two, and sometimes up to the age of four, children are often unable to use a spacer correctly. Most over-fives can learn to use a DPI or breath-actuated inhaler, however, and children aged ten to twelve years should be able to manage an MDI. You can encourage younger children to use a spacer in several ways, as follows.

- If your child is under two years, use a spacer and mask.
- Stroke your child's cheek gently with the mask so that he or she becomes used to the sensation.

- When a mask/spacer combination is used, the valve must be open all the time, so hold the Nebuhaler vertically or the Volumatic at an angle, until you hear a click and the mist containing the medicine emerges from the bottom of the chamber.
- Children inhale after crying. If your child becomes tearful, do not be tempted to unhook the equipment but keep the mask over his or her face until the medicine has been delivered.
- You could administer the medication when your child is asleep to avoid distress.
- Children over two can be taught to use the spacer by practising without pressing the inhaler.
- Decorate the spacer with stickers to make it look more appealing.
- Let your child hold and play with the spacer. Allowing him or her to blow into the spacer is not going to damage it.

For younger children, one alternative is the Babyhaler. This is a small-volume spacer – about half the size of adult spacers – that the baby empties in five to ten breaths. A silicone mask fits over the baby's face, which reduces leakage. The Babyhaler is easy to operate. In an emergency only, you could take a large disposable coffee cup and cut a hole in the bottom, of a size that snugly fits the inhaler mouthpiece. The open end of the cup can then be placed over the baby's face – rather like a mask – and the inhaler actuated through the hole.

How to use a spacer correctly

- Shake the MDI.
- Fit the MDI into a hole at the other end of the spacer from the mouthpiece.
- Press the inhaler.
- Breathe in slowly and steadily through the mouthpiece in one breath. Unlike using an MDI alone, you do not have to time this exactly and can breathe in for up to ten seconds (the sooner the better, though).
- If you feel breathless, breathe as comfortably as possible.
- Actuate the inhaler again when you need to.
- Take shallow breaths in and out half a dozen times.

You may need to service your spacer once a week. Wash it in warm water and mild detergent, rinse it and leave it to dry. Do not wipe it dry – this can lead to a build-up of static electricity, so particles of drug are more likely to stick to the inside and less will reach your lungs. It is worth washing a new spacer before you use it for the first time, to discharge any static electricity left over from the manufacturing process. You should replace a large-volume spacer every six months or so.

Nebulisers

Nebulisers allow people to inhale large amounts of their asthma drug with little effort. They are used either in emergencies, under medical supervision, or to treat people with severe asthma. Nebulisers are about the size of a small briefcase and use ultrasound or compressed air or oxygen to force drug solutions through a narrow hole. This creates a fine mist of tiny droplets, which the person inhales through a facemask or mouthpiece. The small size of the droplets enables them to penetrate deep into the lung. Nebulisers can be used by people of all ages to administer a wide range of drugs, including anti-inflammatories, bronchodilators and anticholinergics.

Make sure your doctor offers written instructions on how to use and maintain the nebuliser. It's worth remembering that using a nebuliser can be time-consuming: nebulisers may take 20 minutes to run a 2.5 to 4 ml solution – the usual quantity. You should inhale all the contents and the nebuliser should be allowed to run dry – signalled by a spluttering sound. Rinsing your mouth and face after using a nebuliser can help limit side-effects. Using a mouthpiece rather than a mask can reduce facial irritation and improve the amount of the dose that gets to your lungs.

Most doctors now carry nebulisers for emergencies. But large-volume spacers (see above) are often just as effective as a nebuliser and in an emergency can be used to deliver the same dose of bronchodilator. In addition to 'rescue' medication delivery, other uses include nebulised steroid – sometimes given if inhaled steroids fail to control symptoms – although this should not be seen as an alternative to a course of oral steroids. Less commonly, nebulisers are used for people unable to use inhaler devices adequately.

There is a danger of becoming over-reliant on a nebuliser. This is because they can mask the symptoms of asthma and delay life-saving anti-inflammatory treatment. Doctors usually advise parents to seek medical help if a child needs nebulised bronchodilators more than every three or four hours. Using a nebuliser more than every two hours suggests that the child is experiencing a severe attack and needs urgent medical help. It is advisable for anyone requiring a nebuliser to see a respiratory specialist regularly.

Chapter summary

A wide variety of drugs and delivery devices are available to treat asthma. You should think of the inhaler and the drug as working together. The range of drugs, used along with the 'stepped care' approach to asthma management, controls the symptoms of the vast majority of people with asthma.

Chapter 8

Allergic eczema and other skin problems

This chapter looks at the allergic skin disorder atopic dermatitis – also called allergic eczema – and three related conditions: contact dermatitis, urticaria ('hives') and angioedema. Because atopic dermatitis, contact dermatitis and urticaria can cause similar symptoms, these skin disorders are often lumped together as 'eczema' or dermatitis. In fact, they show important differences – which may affect treatment.

All these skin diseases can be unpleasant and, in severe cases, may be disfiguring or dangerous. Angioedema (a swelling of tissues below the skin) for example, can be a symptom of anaphylaxis (see Chapter 4). And because these conditions affect the skin, people cannot hide their symptoms and can face prejudice and misunderstanding – for example, that the disease is contagious. Children may endure bullying and teasing in changing rooms or at the swimming pool. Fortunately, a combination of modern medicines and lifestyle changes can control most cases of allergic and the other forms of dermatitis. So it is worth contacting your doctor in all but the mildest cases of eczema, which you may be able to manage using over-the-counter formulations.

Atopic dermatitis (allergic eczema)

Atopic dermatitis is one of the most common allergic diseases, especially in the industrialised world. Between 10 and 20 per cent of children as well as 1 to 3 per cent of adults develop allergic eczema at some time.[1] People with allergic eczema endure dry, itchy, inflamed skin that can blister, weep, thicken and crack. Symptoms tend to wax and wane from day to day. Atopic dermatitis differs from contact dermatitis (see pages 147–50) in the pattern of the symptoms. The itching – called pruritus – can be severe and often tends to be worse in the early evening and night. As we'll see later, antihistamines can alleviate many cases of itching linked to atopic dermatitis. And certain antihistamines – those that cause sedation as a side-effect – can help you sleep. Doctors use skin prick and patch testing (see Chapter 3) to aid in the diagnosis of allergic eczema as well as to try to identify the cause.

In some cases, atopic dermatitis causes rashes that affect just small areas of skin. In the most serious cases, however, the whole body may be involved. To a certain extent, the symptom pattern depends on the person's age. For instance, adults usually develop allergic eczema on the insides and backs of the elbows, the backs of the knees and the hands. Young children tend to develop the rash on the face. But these are not 'hard and fast' differences.

Atopic dermatitis usually emerges in childhood. Indeed, in around 80 per cent of people with allergic eczema, symptoms emerge by their first birthday. In 95 per cent of cases, atopic dermatitis arises during the first five years of life. Nevertheless, dermatologists worldwide are seeing an increasing number of adults who develop allergic eczema for the first time.[2]

Many atopic dermatitis sufferers, then, are too young to understand their disease and its treatment. For instance, they may exacerbate their condition by scratching. (They often can't help this, so shouldn't be scolded.) They may be unable to sleep and make constant demands on their parents – which can leave the entire family tired and irritable. While this can be a difficult time for the children concerned as well as their parents, appropriate treatment is able to effectively control most cases of allergic eczema. Around 60 per cent of cases are mild. Moreover, around half the number of children with atopic dermatitis improve by school age and around 90 per cent of cases resolve during adolescence.[2] Nevertheless, some people with atopic dermatitis experience outbreaks for the rest of their lives.

What causes atopic dermatitis?
Although atopic dermatitis is an allergic disease, we still have much to learn about the exact mechanisms that cause the skin symptoms.

Atopic dermatitis is likely to arise from the interaction of several factors.[3] Increased levels of IgE antibodies and Th_2-cells (both involved in the 'immune cascade' described in Chapter 1) seem to trigger the inflammation and contribute to chronic (long-lasting) atopic dermatitis in between 70 and 80 per cent of cases.[4]

The other 20 or 30 per cent of people with the disease suffer from so-called 'intrinsic' atopic dermatitis. Although an allergic condition, 'intrinsic' atopic dermatitis does not seem to be mediated by IgE. The causes of intrinsic atopic dermatitis are even less well understood than the better-studied IgE-mediated form. However, people with the two forms seem to share at least one set of genes. This offers a starting point for studies into intrinsic atopic dermatitis.

Some genetic factors increase the risk of developing atopic diseases in general. But some seem to specifically increase the risk of developing allergic eczema. For example, the children of parents with atopic dermatitis seem to be more likely to develop allergic eczema than the offspring of parents with asthma or allergic rhinitis.[4]

As with the other common atopic conditions, such as asthma and hay fever, the number of people with allergic eczema in the industrialised world has increased markedly over recent years: between two- and threefold in the last three decades. Again, the reasons are not fully understood. But some researchers consider that the hygiene hypothesis (see Chapter 1) is, perhaps, the most compelling explanation for this dramatic rise.[2] This theory is supported by the fact that atopic dermatitis tends to be less common in predominately rural countries.

It is clear that a multitude of factors can exacerbate atopic dermatitis (see box opposite). Many people report, for instance, that stress makes their allergic eczema worse. Stress can alter the release of hormones released from the adrenal gland, some of which act as natural anti-inflammatories. Stress may limit the production of these natural anti-inflammatory hormones. This could trigger a resurgence in the inflammatory reaction that underlies the eczema.

Sometimes, a combination of atopy (a genetic predisposition to developing certain allergies) and other mechanisms can lead to the symptoms. For example, chemical irritants can exacerbate the allergic symptoms (see 'Contact dermatitis', later in this chapter).

There also seems to be a considerable overlap between atopic dermatitis and food allergies (see Chapter 11). Indeed, about a third of infants and children with moderate to severe atopic dermatitis have a food allergy.[5] As we will see in Chapter 11, egg, milk, wheat, soy and peanut seem to be the most common causes of food-related atopic dermatitis. But identifying the food trigger can be time-consuming and difficult, especially because, as we saw in Chapter 2, people can cross-react to different allergens.

The overlap with other allergic diseases isn't confined to food allergies. For example, children with atopic dermatitis are at least three times more likely to develop asthma than other children. And between 30 and 50 per cent of people with atopic dermatitis respond to aeroallergens – such as house dust mites, pollen from weeds, animal danders and moulds – when applied under a patch.[4] (Although as we saw in Chapter 3, no diagnostic test is infallible – so this doesn't necessarily mean that these allergens caused the allergic eczema.) Exposure to these common aeroallergens is one reason why asthma, rhinitis and atopic dermatitis overlap, but the atopic diseases are also linked on a more fundamental immunological level, as we saw in Chapter 1.

Factors that can exacerbate atopic dermatitis

- Soaps, laundry detergents, perfumes and other irritants.
- Smoke.
- Alcohol and astringents in toiletries – these can worsen dry skin.
- Wool and 'scratchy' or abrasive materials – so it's a good idea to wear cotton.
- Excessive sweating – so swimming may be a better form of exercise than, for example, football. But make sure that you use emollients (skin creams) afterwards, as the chlorine can exacerbate atopic dermatitis.
- Heat. This worsens the condition, partly by increasing sweating.
- Low humidity. For this reason central heating can make skin dry and itchy – so ensure the house is well ventilated.
- Emotional stress: try the relaxation approaches suggested in Chapter 13.

Treatment of atopic dermatitis

Currently, atopic dermatitis cannot be cured (although, as mentioned earlier, many children seem to grow out of the condition.) Nevertheless, finding the correct treatment from the range of drugs available, along with addressing the exacerbating factors outlined in the box above and the lifestyle factors in the box on pages 146–7 should control symptoms in most people.

Needless to say, you should avoid trigger factors as far as practicable. Chapter 2 offers some suggestions to help you limit your exposure to allergens. Some researchers have noted that prolonged efforts to reduce levels of house dust mites (we discussed some strategies to achieve this in Chapter 2) can improve atopic dermatitis in some people.[4] But, to avoid the allergen that is triggering your eczema, you obviously need first to identify it. (Trying to reduce dust mite levels when you're allergic to pollen is a futile and expensive endeavour.) So talk to your doctor, who will be able to suggest appropriate tests.

Emollients

If allergen avoidance fails to adequately control your symptoms, emollients – preparations that help keep the skin moist – will be the mainstay of your atopic dermatitis management. You will use emollients alongside the other treatments outlined below. A layer in the skin called the stratum corneum helps keep skin smooth and flexible by binding water. Emollients hydrate the stratum corneum, making the skin softer and more pliant. Emollients are also anti-inflammatory and often offer some, albeit short-lived, relief from irritation. Emollient formulations are often 'surprisingly complex and sophisticated'.[6] They are certainly effective.

In general, emollients are formulated as either oils or creams. Adding oil emollients to the bath removes crusty skin scales and moisturises the skin. Applying cream emollients directly to the skin after a bath can alleviate the eczema symptoms. You should also apply cream emollients before and after swimming in a pool, as chlorine tends to exacerbate allergic eczema. You should try to remember to apply cream emollients in the direction of hair growth. And you may have to try several emollients before finding one you (or your child) prefer. Fortunately, there is a huge range available. So talk to your doctor or pharmacist.

Antihistamines

If emollients don't control your symptoms, your doctor can suggest a number of other treatments. For example, antihistamine tablets may relieve itching. (Although inflammatory mediators – see Chapter 1 – other than histamine can be responsible for the itching. So antihistamines might not always be effective.) In 2002 the *Drug and Therapeutics Bulletin* (*DTB*)[7] concluded that there is little to choose between the antihistamines in terms of their clinical effectiveness.

Some antihistamines – such as chlorphenamine (Piriton), promethazine (e.g. Phenergan) and clemastine (Tavegil) – cause drowsiness in 10 to 50 per cent of people who take them. This can be a great benefit if you find the itching keeps you awake at night. On the other hand, you should never drive or operate machinery if you find that antihistamine tablets – or any other drug for that matter – make you sleepy, even if it is the morning after you've taken the drug.

Newer antihistamine tablets – such as cetirizine (Zirtek), loratadine (Clarityn) and acrivastine (Benadryl) – are much less likely to lead to sedation and so can be used to relieve itchy skin throughout the day. So doctors may prescribe non-sedative antihistamine tablets for the day and sedative antihistamines at night to aid sleep. *DTB*[7] comments that up to 23 per cent of people find that the newer drugs still make them a bit drowsy – so it is important to pay attention to how you feel. You should not drink alcohol while taking either sedative or non-sedative antihistamine tablets.

Topical steroids

Topical steroids – creams and ointments – are highly effective in relieving the symptoms of atopic dermatitis, such as when the disease flares up. (A topical drug is one you apply to the outside of the body, for example, to the skin.) Steroid ointments are especially useful for dry, scaly skin. In many cases, a topical steroid can resolve the eczema symptoms. However, the rash may come back if you stop using the steroid.

Although they are highly effective, topical steroids can cause a number of side-effects. In 2003, *DTB*[8] commented that mild or moderately potent steroids (see table on page 148) control eczema in most people. When used correctly, these 'very rarely' cause side-

Ways to alleviate atopic dermatitis

You can take several steps to make life more bearable if you or your child has atopic dermatitis.

- Shower in warm, rather than hot, water once a day for less than 10 minutes. Small children with atopic dermatitis should have short baths.
- Pat the skin dry with a soft towel. Try to avoid rubbing your skin.
- Use a moisturiser – ask your doctor or pharmacist for an appropriate formulation. This acts in a similar way to emollients. You might find that you need to use the moisturiser several times a day.
- Drink lots of water, which helps keep the stratum corneum (a skin layer) hydrated.
- Run clothes through two rinse cycles in the washing machine to remove as much washing powder as possible. Detergents can act as irritants, which may exacerbate the allergen's effects.
- Wear gloves when you work with cleaning products and other chemicals. Note, however, that rubber gloves may not block all allergens. Furthermore, latex can cause allergies (see Chapter 2) – at work you could seek advice from your Health and Safety Officer.

effects. However, children tend to be especially vulnerable to developing these reactions, which include:

- skin thinning
- striae – changes to the skin that resemble 'stretch marks'
- mild changes in skin pigmentation
- acne, which can occur wherever steroids are applied. This is one reason why steroids more potent than 1 per cent hydrocortisone (see table on page 148) should not be used on the face
- side-effects elsewhere in the body (see Chapter 7). This is a particular problem when you apply potent steroids to large areas of skin.

Sometimes, the side-effects disappear when you stop using the steroid. But some side-effects, such as some cases of skin thinning

- Some people with atopic dermatitis find that oatmeal bath products make their skin less itchy.
- Wear loose underwear and clothes made of cotton and other natural materials.
- Wash new clothes before wearing them. The material may retain chemicals used in its manufacture.
- If itching is a problem and you find that you scratch, cut your fingernails short and wear cotton gloves at night. And during the day, try to keep your hands busy! Idle hands often scratch.
- It may be worth changing your bubble bath or washing powder. Sometimes, this can be enough to make the atopic dermatitis disappear. More commonly, irritant reactions to these detergents may exacerbate the allergen's effects (see 'Contact dermatitis' on page 149).
- Minimising stress can also help relieve the discomfort associated with eczema, or the distress associated by living with a child suffering from eczema. Try following the suggestions in *The Which? Guide to Managing Stress* or the relaxation techniques in Chapter 13.
- Some people also report benefiting from complementary therapies, including Chinese herbalism. We'll look at these again in Chapter 13.

and striae, may never resolve. So you should apply the mildest steroid that controls your symptoms, to the smallest areas possible for the shortest possible time.

Clearly, it is important to ensure that you use the correct dose of topical steroids. It is easy to under-dose with creams and ointments – for example, by spreading the drug too thinly. The easiest way to ensure you apply sufficient steroid is to ask your doctor for the dose in 'fingertip units'. (The package insert may also give the dose in fingertip units.) This is the amount of steroid cream or ointment that, when expelled from the tube, covers from the tip of the adult index finger to the first crease. A fingertip unit is roughly equivalent to about 500mg and should be enough to cover an area twice that of the flat adult hand.

The potency of different topical steroids	
Potency	**Example**
mild	hydrocortisone 1%
moderate	clobetasone butyrate 0.05%
potent	betamethasone valerate 0.1%, hydrocortisone butyrate 0.1%
very potent	clobetasol propionate 0.05%

Other treatments

If atopic dermatitis does not respond adequately to the treatments outlined above, your GP may refer you to a dermatologist, who can try stronger drugs, including cyclosporine (also spelt ciclosporin; brand names Neoral, Sandimmun and SangCya), a tablet, as well as the topical drugs pimecrolimus (Elidel) and tacrolimus (Protopic). These drugs dampen the immune system.

Tacrolimus, for instance, inhibits several key cells involved in atopic dermatitis, including T-cells and mast cells (see Chapter 1). Tacrolimus ointment, unlike topical steroids, does not seem to cause skin thinning. However, about half of the people using it develop a transitory burning sensation, itching or erythema (patchy redness) at the application site. There is a theoretical risk that long-term use of tacrolimus could, because it suppresses the immune system, increase the risk of skin cancer or an infection, but this needs further investigation.[9] Tacrolimus ointment can also sometimes cause infections at the application site and severe reactions to sunlight.

In people with severe atopic dermatitis, these immunosuppressants can be highly effective. But cyclosporine – also used to help prevent transplant recipients from rejecting their organs, which gives you an idea of its potency – can cause numerous side-effects, some of which are potentially serious. Tacrolimus ointment is approved for use only when other treatments fail.

The National Eczema Society* can offer further advice and support.

Contact dermatitis

Allergy, chemical irritation or a combination of both can cause contact dermatitis: the symptoms of which, like those of atopic dermatitis, range from a few areas of red rash to cracked weeping skin to – in rare cases – widespread eczema. The itching can be severe and the skin may blister, and in some cases the skin can thicken. Any skin surface that comes into contact with the trigger, which may include aeroallergens, can develop contact dermatitis.

Unlike other forms of eczema, the symptoms of contact dermatitis don't, in general, wax and wane from day to day because, as the name suggests, the person is continually exposed to the trigger. Furthermore, the dermatitis, at least at first, tends to be confined to the area in contact with the trigger, which is usually the hands. However, over time the rash may spread – especially in allergic contact dermatitis.

Contact dermatitis is common, with occupational irritants emerging as the most common cause. Indeed, if the substance is sufficiently aggressive, almost everyone in contact with it will develop contact dermatitis. A report in 2003 by the Royal College of Physicians[10] notes that contact dermatitis accounts for half of all sickness leave. A UK study[11] found that 12.9 people for every 100,000 workers developed occupational contact dermatitis. People employed in manufacturing were the most likely to develop the condition, followed by healthcare workers. Hairdressers, barbers and agriculture workers were also prone to developing occupational contact dermatitis.

In some cases you'll need to undergo patch tests or a challenge test (see Chapter 3) although, as we've seen, these are not infallible. However, some clues could lead you to suspect an occupational irritant. For example, typically, occupational contact dermatitis clears during a two- or three-week break from work, but the eczema usually recurs when the person returns (for example, from holiday). Occasionally, mild eczema may improve over the weekend – but, in general, as mentioned above, the symptoms don't alter markedly from day to day.[12]

Another study[13] has shown that contact dermatitis tends to emerge during the first year in a new job. It can also emerge when a new chemical or process is introduced. Allergies take at least two weeks to develop. This delay reflects the time taken for antibodies to develop. However, strong irritants can produce symptoms within minutes to hours. Weaker irritants may need several cumulative exposures to cause contact dermatitis.

Doctors can distinguish irritant and allergic contact dermatitis by placing a non-irritating concentration of the suspected trigger under a patch (see Chapter 3). Allergies arise following exposure to very low levels of the trigger. So if the person develops a reaction to the low concentration, the symptoms are probably allergic. If a higher concentration is needed to provoke a response, the person probably has irritant contact dermatitis.

Once you suspect, or have confirmed, an occupational substance as the trigger for your eczema, it is clearly important to follow the handling instructions on the chemical. When using protective gloves, remember that rubber does not keep out many allergens and that latex allergies are increasingly common (see Chapter 2). If you are in any doubt about how to handle the chemical in question, or about the protective measures that you need to take, talk to your Health and Safety Officer.

Sometimes people develop irritant contact dermatitis to items of clothing, cosmetics, watches or jewellery. Nickel, perfumes and fragrances are common causes of contact dermatitis. For instance, the nickel in bra clasps can produce local reactions, typically a small outbreak of eczema on the spine. Several drugs, including steroid creams and ointments, can also cause contact dermatitis. (We'll look again at drug-induced allergies in Chapter 12.) So if you develop a rash after starting treatment with a drug, talk to your doctor or pharmacist.

Avoiding the trigger is critical to the management of contact dermatitis. Indeed, although steroid tablets and ointments can help, and antihistamines may alleviate itching, treatment often proves ineffective unless the trigger is removed. In some cases, such as the allergy to nickel in bra straps, identifying the cause can be relatively straightforward. At other times, a patch test will be necessary. Again, if you feel that the symptoms might be caused by an occupational allergen, talk to your Health and Safety Officer and to your GP, who should be able to arrange for the appropriate tests.

Urticaria

Urticaria, also known as 'hives' or nettle rash, can arise following exposure to allergens, producing the classic 'weal and flare' allergic response (see Chapter 1). The usual suspects – such as foods, drugs, animal danders, pollens or latex rubber – are often responsible. In rare cases, food allergies cause chronic (long-lasting) urticaria; in general, they cause rapidly developing symptoms such as, in sensitive people, urticaria around the mouth after eating strawberries or a rash after eating seafood. Often doctors can diagnose such cases of acute (rapid-onset) urticaria, caused by food, based on the person's history and sometimes by using other diagnostic tests (see Chapter 3).[5]

Physical stimuli – such as changes in temperature or pressure, scratching and sunlight – can also lead to weal and flare. Sunlight, for instance, can cause degranulation of mast cells – part of the immune response underlying allergic reactions (see Chapter 1). Changes in the nervous system following a rise in body temperature, emotional stress or exercise can also lead to urticaria.

Sometimes the body seems to generate antibodies to the receptors on mast cells that bind IgE (so-called 'autoimmunity'). The antibodies trigger mast cell degranulation. In other cases, the cause can prove difficult to track down and, more often than not, doctors cannot identify an allergic or physical cause for the urticaria. Such cases are called 'idiopathic urticaria'.

Once the triggers have been identified or idiopathic urticaria diagnosed, antihistamine tablets are the main treatment. Antihistamines may, however, be less effective in people with idiopathic urticaria than the other forms of the condition. The doctor may suggest non-sedative antihistamines for the daytime use. Sedative antihistamines can be used during the night. Some people need oral steroids (see Chapter 7) or, more rarely, immunosuppressants (see page 147).

Angioedema

Angioedema is a swelling of tissue under the layer of fat just below the skin. It can occur alone or with urticaria, hay fever, or food or drug allergy. It may also be a symptom of anaphylaxis (see Chapter 4) and, as this suggests, angioedema can be serious. For instance, angioedema affecting the tongue and larynx (voice box) can lead to breathlessness or difficulty in speaking.

The Royal College of Physicians report[10] suggests that an allergist should manage people suffering from angioedema – especially if severe. As with urticaria, oral antihistamines are the main treatment for angioedema. Sometimes the person may need high doses of these drugs. And, again, the doctor may combine non-sedative and sedative antihistamines or prescribe oral steroids or, more rarely, immunosuppressants.

Chapter summary

Allergic eczema and related skin diseases can be unpleasant and, occasionally, either disfiguring or potentially serious. In some cases, these conditions seem to arise through the IgE-mediated route that underlies the other classic atopic diseases. In others, a different immune mechanism or a direct chemical irritation seems to cause the symptoms. And sometimes the cause can be a mix of atopy and other mechanisms. Chemical irritation can exacerbate atopic dermatitis, for example. Currently, other than by avoiding the trigger, allergic and other forms of eczema cannot be cured. But a combination of lifestyle changes and modern medicines control symptoms in most people.

Chapter 9

Hay fever and other forms of rhinitis

You see them everywhere in the spring and summer: people sneezing, rubbing their noses or dabbing tears from their eyes. It's the hay fever season. For millions of people the onset of summer heralds weeks or months of discomfort. Fortunately, you can take medicines and other steps to keep the symptoms under control.

Hay fever is a misnomer. Hay doesn't trigger rhinitis – inflammation of the lining of the nose – and you don't develop a fever (although some people break out in a cold sweat). Nevertheless, for many, allergic rhinitis causes considerable distress. Although it is common, the condition isn't trivial. A report in 2003 by the Royal College of Physicians[1] comments that rhinitis can, in some cases, undermine quality of life as severely as asthma.

Doctors first recognised hay fever – or seasonal allergic rhinitis – as a disease in 1819. But the cause of this summer catarrh – a 'periodal affection of the chest and eyes' – remained a mystery for several years. Some doctors believed that ozone could trigger the condition. (We now know that ozone can exacerbate many allergic diseases, including rhinitis.) Others thought that the odour given off by plants caused the symptoms. Still others believed that dust from beaten carpets and from the roads led to rhinitis. Today, we recognise, of course, that the house dust mite is a significant allergen – triggering, in addition to asthma and eczema – perennial rhinitis.

Other allergens that can trigger rhinitis include airborne particles containing latex, flour dust and animal dander (dead skin and hair). Several non-allergic triggers – such as cigarette smoke – can also exacerbate symptoms. But classic 'hay fever' is, of course, caused by pollen. As we saw in Chapter 2, grass is the most common source of allergenic pollen. Ninety-five per cent of hay fever sufferers are allergic to grass pollen. If someone is allergic to more than one pollen, his or her hay fever season can extend for many months. We looked at the pollen seasons for different plants and at other allergenic triggers in Chapter 2. In this chapter, we'll look at the symptoms of allergic rhinitis and the best way to treat this common condition.

Symptoms of allergic rhinitis

Allergic rhinitis is very, very common – which may be one reason why both sufferers with mild symptoms and doctors sometimes trivialise the complaint. Indeed, between a tenth and a quarter of the world's population experience allergic rhinitis.[2] However, the disease is much more common in Western countries than in predominately rural areas of the world. Furthermore, as with other atopic diseases, the number of people with hay fever is rising rapidly in the industrialised world – increasing between two- and threefold over the last 20 to 30 years.[1] The causes of the rise are not fully understood, but it seems likely that the hygiene hypothesis (see Chapter 1) might be the best explanation. And, as discussed below, asthma and allergic rhinitis are intimately linked. Certainly, allergic rhinitis is more common in children than in adults, affecting up to 40 per cent of children.[3]

Essentially, allergic rhinitis is a hypersensitivity of the nose to triggers and allergens that most people find innocuous. In many cases, the 'immune cascade' discussed in Chapter 1 causes the symptoms. But as we have seen, a number of non-allergic triggers can exacerbate the condition. Certain other diseases can also lead to rhinitis – see box on page 157.

In mild cases, people might feel just an itch or slight irritation of the mucous membranes. Many people also develop sore, red eyes – a condition called allergic conjunctivitis. (Chapter 10 considers allergic conjunctivitis and its treatment in more detail. You should read these two chapters together.) The nose feels stuffy; people endure attacks of severe sneezing and produce copious amounts of a watery discharge from their nose (rhinorrhea).

Occasionally, rhinitis sufferers can break into a cold sweat. In some cases – for example, when the allergen is the house dust mite or animal dander (see Chapter 2) – the allergy symptoms can disturb sleep, leading to daytime fatigue and somnolence. As a result, allergic rhinitis can impair performance at school or work. (This is bad news for sufferers sitting exams, which are often held at the height of the hay fever season.) The symptoms abate only when exposure to the allergen ceases.

But some researchers note that allergic inflammation alone cannot explain the chronic (persistent) nature of rhinitis. They suggest that the inflammation can change the cells lining the upper airway (the epithelium), which leads to the condition becoming chronic.[2] (This is similar to 'remodelling' in asthma – see Chapter 5) Others point out that mast cell degranulation and the recruitment of cells involved in the late-phase allergic reaction – see Chapter 1 – can lead to marked oedema (swelling), tissue damage and chronic inflammation.[4] As a result, polyps – small, non-cancerous growths – eventually develop. Doctors describe this condition as 'nasal polyposis'.

Seasonal or perennial – what's the difference?

Seasonal rhinitis occurs only during the pollen season for the particular allergen (see Chapter 2). But if the allergen is present all year around, the rhinitis could occur for most, or even all, of the year. This is called perennial allergic rhinitis.

House dust mites and pet dander cause most cases of perennial allergic rhinitis, which, like the seasonal form, is very common. In a study[5] of more than 80,000 people taking medicines to treat allergic rhinitis, the prescribing data suggested that 79 per cent showed seasonal symptoms, while in 21 per cent the symptoms were perennial. Allergies underlie all cases of seasonal rhinitis, but cause only about 60 to 70 per cent of perennial cases. The remainder arise from one of the number of other conditions listed in the box on page 158.

Allergic rhinitis and asthma

Apart from the marked impact on quality of life, there is one very good reason why you shouldn't trivialise rhinitis. Doctors recognised decades ago that allergic rhinitis can lead to asthma. Some people develop asthma symptoms in the hay fever season: this form is sometimes called 'hay asthma' or 'summer asthma'. In others, it seems that allergic rhinitis can be the first sign of changes in the respiratory tract that can develop into asthma.

Considerable evidence now suggests that, in many cases, allergic rhinitis and asthma are manifestations of the same underlying disease. For example, doctors discovered during the 1920s that tissues from people with asthma and hay fever showed high levels of eosinophils, a type of white blood cell linked to some allergies. Indeed, people with asthma often develop rhinitis in response to the same allergen. So some scientists think that the difference between rhinitis and asthma is anatomical, rather than immunological.[6] For example, nasal passages may be exposed to higher local levels of pollen and other allergens than the lungs. So perhaps it's not surprising that the immune cascade can begin in the nose before developing in the lungs.

The intimate relationship between the two conditions leads some researchers to suggest that treating allergic rhinitis might prevent asthma. Further studies are needed to confirm how effective such preventative strategies may be. But it seems a logical and promising approach – and is another good reason to ensure that your rhinitis symptoms are effectively treated. That might mean seeing your GP rather than relying on over-the-counter medications, especially if your symptoms are severe or start getting worse.

On the other hand, sometimes concurrent asthma may lead doctors to underestimate the impact of rhinitis. So if you suffer from both it's important to ensure that your doctor appreciates the severity of your rhinitis.

Treatment of allergic rhinitis

Over the years, doctors tried numerous treatments to alleviate hay fever – including oil of chamomile, solutions of adrenaline and methanol, and even snuffs and sprays containing cocaine. Not surprisingly, using cocaine snuffs and sprays led, in some cases, to addiction.

Fortunately, today's medicines offer a number of effective and, in general, well-tolerated treatments for rhinitis. Some of these you can buy over the counter from your local pharmacist. Your GP can also prescribe more effective treatments, often more potent versions of the drugs you can buy from the chemist.

Other causes of rhinitis

Allergic reactions account for most cases of rhinitis. But a number of other diseases can also lead to the condition. For example:

- viral or bacterial infections
- structural abnormalities in the nose's internal shape
- chronic sinusitis – persistent inflammation of the nasal sinuses
- nasal polyps
- hypothyroidism – when people produce inadequate levels of hormones from the thyroid gland. Hormones released by the thyroid gland, which is in the neck, control growth, development and metabolism
- certain drugs, including the combined contraceptive pill, aspirin and beta-blockers. (Beta-blockers are used to manage several diseases, including high blood pressure.) Some of these drugs can trigger an allergic or 'hypersensitivity' reaction (see Chapter 12). However, their biological effects also mean that they can trigger rhinitis through non-allergic mechanisms.

Moreover, allergic rhinitis is often associated with sinusitis and otitis media (glue ear),[3] which are not life-threatening. But if one nostril feels blocked and you expel a bloodstained discharge from either side you should seek medical advice urgently. In rare cases, a cancer in the nose, sinuses or surrounding tissue can cause these symptoms.

As a rule, people who have perennial allergic rhinitis should consult their GP. As the symptoms occur year round, you will need to take treatment long-term and so would benefit from a GP's advice. In addition, a GP can rule out many of the other conditions that can lead to symptoms of rhinitis (see box above) and, where appropriate, refer you for further investigations by specialists.

Two other points are worth remembering. Firstly, most people with hay fever will also need to manage allergic conjunctivitis, which is discussed in Chapter 10. Secondly, there is some scientific evidence that homeopathy (see Chapter 13) could benefit some people with allergic rhinitis. For example, the results of several studies together showed that symptoms of allergic rhinitis improved by an average of 28 per cent among homeopathy users compared to 3 per cent in the placebo group (see page 213).

Allergen avoidance

As with other allergic conditions, allergen avoidance is the first step in managing allergic rhinitis. We looked at some tips to reduce your exposure to common allergens in Chapter 2. However, some allergens prove remarkably resilient. For example, researchers reviewed several studies that examined physical and chemical ways to prevent exposure to house dust mites in the homes of people with perennial allergic rhinitis. In all cases, although levels of the dust mites fell markedly, there was 'little evidence' that clinical symptoms improved. On the other hand, these researchers commented that the studies reviewed involved small numbers of people and were of 'poor quality'.[7] Clearly, more investigation is needed. But a better designed trial also produced somewhat negative results. In this case, bedding covers that are impermeable to dust mites reduced levels of the allergen. But, again, the 279 people with allergic rhinitis who were sensitised to dust mites did not show any improvement in their symptoms.[8]

You could certainly try dust mite avoidance – and it might work for you. It might be especially appropriate if skin prick tests suggest that you could be allergic to dust mites. But you should be aware that you will almost certainly need to employ several measures to reduce your exposure to dust mites (see Chapter 2 for further advice) – covers or sprays alone may not be sufficient. And you're likely to need to take medication as well. It's certainly worth keeping a record of your symptoms to help identify the trigger, and so make sure that you're not wasting your time and money. See Chapter 3 for advice on keeping an allergy diary.

Intranasal steroids

If used regularly, most people find that intranasal corticosteroids are the most effective treatment for allergic rhinitis (see box on page 160). Several intranasal steroids are currently available, as drops or sprays, from either chemists or your GP (who can prescribe higher doses and longer treatment courses). The main ones are beclomethasone (also spelled beclometasone – brands include

Beclogen, Beconase and Nasobec) fluticasone (Flixonase) and budesonide (Rhinocort), and they seem to differ little in their effectiveness. You take beclomethasone nasal spray between two and four times a day, depending on the severity of your symptoms; budesonide and fluticasone are taken once or twice daily. Intranasal steroids reduce the underlying inflammation of rhinitis (see Chapter 7 for more about how steroids work) so reduce symptoms – the nasal blockage, discharge, sneezing, itching and dripping. If taken regularly, intranasal steroids reduce the likelihood that allergic rhinitis will develop when you are exposed to the allergen. However, the effects of steroids can take several days to fully emerge.

One study[9] found that budesonide reduced nasal congestion and improved sleep. As a result, the subjects reported less tiredness during the day. However, intranasal steroids can cause several side-effects, including dryness and irritation of the nose and throat, nosebleeds, headaches and changes in smell and taste. More rarely, they can lead to glaucoma, an increase in the pressure inside the eye. This can damage the delicate light-sensitive retina at the back of the eye.

Furthermore, using high doses of intranasal steroids for long periods – for example, to treat severe perennial rhinitis – can mean enough of the drug gets in the bloodstream to cause systemic side-effects (effects elsewhere in the body – see Chapter 7). The risk of systemic side-effects seems to be greater with drops than sprays. This may reflect the fact that people are more likely to use drops incorrectly. So it is very important to follow the dosing instructions given to you by the doctor and on the package insert. If you are in any doubt how to use the medicine, speak to your local pharmacist or doctor.

The risk of side-effects – especially the systemic adverse effects – means that you shouldn't use intranasal steroids for more than three months without consulting a doctor. Furthermore, intranasal steroids should not be used in people under the age of 18, unless under medical supervision.

Because long-term use of high-dose steroids may, in some cases, retard growth, children undergoing prolonged treatment with intranasal steroids should have their height measured regularly by a doctor or nurse. While this is prudent, the chance of steroid use affecting growth seems relatively low. In one study,[10] 78 children, received 256 to 400 mcg intranasal budesonide daily for between one and two years. No effects on growth were evident – despite the duration of the treatment.

Antihistamines

Antihistamines, which specifically block the effects of the inflammatory mediator histamine (see Chapter 1), are especially effective against the early-phase rhinitis symptoms, such as dripping nose, sneezing and itching. They tend to be less effective against the late-phase reactions, such as blocked and congested nasal passages, which are caused by inflammatory mediators other than histamine. Antihistamines are available as nose drops or tablets; the latter tend to be more effective than the former. Antihistamines work more rapidly than nasal steroids.

When used according to the prescription or manufacturer's instructions, antihistamines rarely cause serious side-effects. But some antihistamines, especially alimemazine (Rhinolast, Aller-eze) – also called trimeprazine – commonly cause sedation and drowsiness. Newer antihistamines are less likely to cause sedation

---

Steroids or antihistamines?

So how do the two main treatments for allergic rhinitis compare? One review of 16 studies[11] found that intranasal steroids were more effective than oral antihistamines against nasal blockage, discharge, sneezing, itching and dripping. Intranasal steroids also reduced the total number and severity of symptoms to a greater extent than antihistamines. But both treatments alleviated eye symptoms or nasal discomfort to a similar extent. The researchers suggested that intranasal steroids should be the treatment of choice for allergic rhinitis. Oral antihistamines can be a useful treatment in addition to steroids for eye symptoms or nasal itching when steroids alone are not effective. It's also worth remembering that, because antihistamines work more rapidly than steroids, they may alleviate many of the symptoms while the steroids reduce the underlying inflammation.

(see page 145). Nevertheless, if you feel tired after using any antihistamine you should not drive or operate machinery. You should also avoid alcohol while taking antihistamines, because this can increase the risk of sedation. And you should always ensure that the pharmacist, doctor or nurse knows of any other medications you are taking, either bought over the counter or on prescription.

Other side-effects of antihistamines include headache, dry mouth, blurred vision, gastrointestinal disturbances, palpitations, allergic reactions (see Chapter 12), dizziness, confusion and sleep disturbances. But in general, these adverse reactions are unusual.

Decongestants

Decongestants, as their name suggests, alleviate nasal congestion. This congestion arises when membranes and tissues inside the nose swell so much that they impede the airflow. Decongestants relax the airways. This makes breathing easier, although these drugs have little effect on the blockage itself. Many of these are available over the counter. Indeed, the decongestants are not available on NHS prescription.

Some decongestants – such as pseudoephedrine (e.g. Galpseud, Sudafed) – are taken orally. Nasal decongestants (nose drops and sprays) include ipratropium (Rinatec) and xylometazoline (e.g. Otraspray, Otrivine). Some decongestants are also available combined with antihistamines. These may, as mentioned above, cause drowsiness or impair your ability to operate machinery.

It's probably best to stick to nasal decongestants if possible, as these tend to cause fewer adverse reactions than the oral forms. Decongestants are mild stimulants, although pseudoephedrine may cause fewer such effects than some of the others. The higher concentrations in the blood with oral decongestants mean that they can cause insomnia, restlessness, rapid heartbeat, urinary retention and increased blood pressure. They can exacerbate the following conditions, and so should be used carefully in these cases:

- high blood pressure
- diabetes
- hyperthyroidism – an overactive thyroid gland

- raised intraocular pressure – the pressure inside the eye. Raised intraocular pressure can damage the delicate light-sensitive retina at the back of the eye, leading to glaucoma
- prostate hypertrophy – an enlargement of the prostate gland in men (see Glossary)
- liver and kidney disease.

It's probably best for everyone to avoid formulations containing phenylpropanolamine, which is linked to an increased risk of haemorrhagic stroke – caused when a blood vessel in the brain bursts. Phenylpropanolamine is included in several cough and decongestant preparations. (Decongestants also alleviate cold symptoms.) So it is worth asking the pharmacist whether the formulation contains phenylpropanolamine.

You should really check with your doctor before using decongestants, especially if you think you could have one of the above diseases. Indeed, everyone should have their blood pressure checked regularly. If you haven't had it measured for a while, you should consider asking your GP or nurse to take a measurement before starting treatment with decongestants.

Using decongestants, especially nasal formulations, can lead to 'rebound' congestion when you stop taking them, as well as resistance. In other words, the congestion gets worse while the drug becomes less effective. Therefore you shouldn't use decongestants for more than a week. And try to allow at least a fortnight between courses of treatment. If you need to use more than a couple of courses over a year, it is probably worth seeing your GP.

Decongestants can also interact with other drugs, including monoamine oxidase inhibitors, one of a number of drugs used to treat depression. So it is important to tell your pharmacist, doctor or nurse about any medicine you are taking. Despite these limitations, however, decongestants can be useful in the short term, to get you through an especially difficult patch.

Sodium cromoglycate

Sodium cromoglycate (also spelled cromoglicate) is a mast cell stabiliser – in other words, it stops mast cells from releasing histamine (see Chapter 1). Available as eye drops and nasal sprays, sodium cromoglycate relieves some symptoms of allergic rhinitis.

It's especially effective for red, itchy eyes (see Chapter 10). But sodium cromoglycate does not relieve nasal congestion. It has only a short duration of action and so needs to be taken regularly – depending on the formulation, you may need to administer the drug into each nostril between two and six times a day. Sodium cromoglycate causes few side-effects, although some people experience irritation in their nose.

Immunotherapy

Immunotherapy, also called desensitisation, switches off the response to the allergen and is often highly effective in seasonal allergic rhinitis. (See page 19 for more details.) Desensitisation might also be effective against allergies triggered by cat dander and house dust mites, as well as in perennial allergic rhinitis. But the Royal College of Physicians report[1] mentioned earlier suggests that more studies in these allergies need to be performed to fully assess the benefits. Immunotherapy does not seem to alleviate non-allergic forms of rhinitis, which are not caused by a hypersensitive immune system.

Surgery

If drug treatments fail to adequately control rhinitis symptoms, surgery may help. For example, as we saw earlier, chronic inflammation caused by allergies can lead to nasal polyps. Surgeons can remove the polyps. Depending on the technique, surgery prevents recurrence in between 60 and 75 per cent of people with nasal polyposis. On average, these people remain free of polyps for between three and four years. Only between 2 and 6 per cent of people develop serious complications following an operation for nasal polyposis.[4] In some cases, surgeons also cut the nerves that contribute to some of the symptoms of rhinitis, such as sneezing.

An alternative approach to rhinitis symptoms uses a small electrode to apply a pulse of radiofrequency energy to tissues in the nose. This injures the cells. The resulting scar tissue shrinks the inflamed tissue. One study[12] found that radiofrequency surgery improved at least one symptom of allergic rhinitis in 91 per cent of people who did not respond adequately to drugs. A year later, the severity of nasal obstruction, rhinorrhea and sneezing improved by 64, 55 and 51 per cent respectively. The severity of itchy nose and eyes improved by 51 and 47 per cent respectively. There are several other surgical procedures available for rhinitis, and a referral to an Ear, Nose and Throat surgeon can help decide which approach is best for you.

Chapter summary

Allergic rhinitis – a hypersensitivity of the nose – is becoming increasingly common, especially among children. Allergic rhinitis and asthma are often manifestations of the same underlying disease. Symptoms of rhinitis can range from an itching or slight irritation of the mucous membranes to severe allergic conjunctivitis, prolonged attacks of sneezing, nasal blockage and copious nasal discharge. Seasonal allergic rhinitis occurs only during the hay fever season for the particular allergen; perennial allergic rhinitis occurs throughout the year. Drugs from the chemist or your GP can alleviate the symptoms. If these fail, immunotherapy or surgery might help.

Chapter 10

Allergic conjunctivitis

Your conjunctiva is a thin layer of cells that covers the whites of your eyes and extends around the insides of your eyelids. Conjunctivitis is an inflammation of this thin lining. Several diseases can cause conjunctival symptoms. In some cases – allergic conjunctivitis, for instance – both eyes are usually affected. Infections, on the other hand, may cause symptoms in only one eye.

As with other allergic diseases, numerous triggers can cause conjunctivitis. Pollen, for example, can cause seasonal allergic conjunctivitis. This occurs only during the season for the particular allergen. House dust mites, moulds and other indoor allergens may trigger perennial allergic conjunctivitis. See Chapter 2 for more about the pollen seasons for different plants and about other allergens. Conjunctivitis can also be a symptom of allergic rhinitis (see Chapter 9). And atopic keratoconjunctivitis (which we'll return to later) arises when atopic dermatitis (allergic eczema – see Chapter 8) affects the eye.

Several non-allergic triggers, as well as some diseases, can also lead to conjunctivitis. These include the following.

- Cosmetics.
- Contact lenses (see box on page 167).
- Dry eyes. A thin film of tears covers the conjunctiva. Dry eyes occur when production of this tear film is inadequate.
- Foreign bodies, such as dust, grit or sand.
- Glaucoma, which is caused by a build-up of pressure in the eye. This increased pressure damages the light-sensitive nerves that make up the retina at the back of the eye. Untreated glaucoma can lead to blindness.
- Styes, caused by swollen glands on the edge of the eyelid. These are usually caused by bacterial infections.
- Bacterial or viral infections.

If you are worried about any eye symptoms, you should see your GP or optician. If an optician thinks you need medication, he or she will tell you to see your GP. Make sure the optician gives you a letter describing his or her findings. In some cases, a GP may refer you to an optician before making the final decision about treatment.

The eye's defences

As the above suggests, potential causes of allergic and other forms of conjunctivitis are everywhere. So it's not surprising that the eye has evolved numerous defence mechanisms.

- Blinking and tear flow help wash allergens and other foreign bodies from the eye (this increased tear production – or 'lacrimation' – causes the streaming eyes common among hay fever sufferers)
- Tears contain several proteins that protect the eye from allergens, as well as natural antibiotics that reduce the risk of infection
- The eyelids and eyelashes help keep the eye moist as well as protecting the conjunctiva from larger particles.

If the allergen or infection breaches these 'non-specific' defences, white blood cells swing into action (see Chapter 1). For example, the 'cocktail' of inflammatory mediators released from mast cells plays a central role in driving signs and symptoms of allergic conjunctivitis, including itching, red eyes and lacrimation. Indeed, the number of mast cells in the conjunctiva of allergic people increases threefold during the allergy season compared with the winter months.[1]

Our eyes can respond to the various invaders with several different immune-based reactions. In general, severe inflammation and serious diseases rarely affect the eyes – which illustrates the effectiveness of our ocular defences. However, the more chronic (long-lasting) and severe forms of conjunctivitis are characterised by persistently high levels of white blood cells,[2] which, by releasing mediators, damage the eye – sometimes irreparably. Fortunately, such cases are rare. For most people, simple treatments can alleviate conjunctival symptoms and avert any long-term problems.

Contact lenses and conjunctivitis

Contact lenses can trigger and exacerbate conjunctivitis through several mechanisms, as follows.[3]

- Wearing contact lenses might make an immune response more likely.
- Contact lenses can absorb some preservatives, cleaning agents and other chemicals used in their care. These chemicals can then gradually leach out and can directly irritate the eye. In a few people, these chemicals trigger non-allergic conjunctivitis or exacerbate allergic eye reactions.
- People wearing contacts – especially the soft lenses – can develop an unpleasant condition known as 'giant papillary conjunctivitis'. So you should see your GP or optician as soon as possible if you experience red eyes, a burning sensation, itching, increased tear production or mucous discharge. The burning sensation associated with giant papillary conjunctivitis tends to be especially noticeable when you move your eye.
- Wearing contacts when you have allergic conjunctivitis can increase the risk of contracting an eye infection. So wear your glasses instead until the symptoms abate.

How common is allergic conjunctivitis?

Conjunctivitis generally is perhaps the most widespread eye disease. But, as mentioned above, it can be triggered by a number of different factors. So how common is the allergic form?

In most cases, allergic conjunctivitis arises during the hay fever season (see Chapter 2). Almost all hay fever sufferers have some associated eye symptoms. This combination of nasal symptoms (see Chapter 9) and conjunctivitis is known as 'rhinoconjunctivitis'. Perhaps one in twelve people with hay fever experiences conjunctivitis alone. One in five experiences conjunctivitis as his or her main symptom. This is illustrated by a study of the pattern of symptoms in 509 hay fever sufferers in Switzerland;[4] almost all – 93.3 per cent – showed conjunctivitis to a greater or lesser extent. In 8 per cent, conjunctivitis was the only hay fever symptom. In around 22 per cent, conjunctivitis was the predominant symptom. Children and adolescents with hay fever seemed especially prone to developing conjunctivitis.

But perennial (year-round) symptoms are also common. For example, a UK study[5] found that 18 per cent – almost one in five – of 27,507 children had had rhinoconjunctivitis in the previous 12 months. A third of the children reported perennial symptoms. Another third reported conjunctivitis between March to September only; the remainder reported symptoms at other times of the year.

The pattern of symptoms can, as we suggested in Chapter 2, help you identify the cause of the allergic conjunctivitis. In this way it might be possible to avoid or at least lessen the impact of the allergen. You can also undergo the non-specific diagnostic tests suggested in Chapter 3.

Symptoms of allergic conjunctivitis

The hallmarks of allergic conjunctivitis are red, watery, itchy eyes. The eyelids may become swollen or puffy. In the vast majority of cases the condition affects both eyes. However, a red, watery eye can also be a symptom of several other diseases: eye infections, for example, can produce broadly similar symptoms. Most of these diseases are unpleasant and some can threaten your sight. So it is important to consult your doctor or optician to ascertain whether you really do have allergic conjunctivitis. Don't rely on self-diagnosis. However, the box opposite offers some clues to identifying whether your eye symptoms are allergic or infective.

Allergic conjunctivitis can take several forms.

Seasonal allergic conjunctivitis
This is also called hay fever conjunctivitis. The symptoms of itching, redness, and watering eyes are confined to the allergen season. It's hard to avoid rubbing the eyes to relieve the itching – but this can exacerbate the eyelid swelling. The eyes appear bloodshot or pink and produce watery or mucous discharge. Seasonal allergic conjunctivitis doesn't usually affect vision.

Recognising infective conjunctivitis

Several clues hint that you might suffer from conjunctivitis caused by an infection – but you should not rely on self-diagnosis.

- The symptoms of infective conjunctivitis tend to emerge between five and twelve days after infection. Initially, at least, the symptoms may appear in only one eye.
- Conjunctivitis caused by infections tends not to itch as intensely as allergic conjunctivitis. In many cases, infective conjunctivitis might not itch at all.
- Infective conjunctivitis can leave the eye feeling as if it is burning or stinging. Some people feel as if there is a foreign body in their eye.
- Some infections lead to the production of copious amounts of discharge. This can lead to the eyelashes becoming 'matted' together with pus. When this dries, overnight for example, it can form a crust. Crusting on the eyelids when you wake in the morning can make opening your eyes difficult.
- Discharge caused by bacterial infection might smell. Viral infections, in contrast, tend to produce a watery discharge.

Whether you think you have allergic or infective conjunctivitis, contact your doctor or optician. Infective conjunctivitis tends to be unpleasant rather than sight threatening. But, nevertheless, viral infections can leave a scar on the cornea (the transparent layer at the front of the eye) for a couple of years. Occasionally, the scarring can impair vision or lead to glare.

Some infections that cause conjunctivitis can be very contagious. So if you or someone in your family suffers from infective conjunctivitis you should ensure that they, and everyone with whom they are in contact, wash their hands with soap often during the day. Try not to touch or rub the infected eyes.

Viral infections tend to last between one and three weeks, depending on the severity. However, in rare cases they persist for longer; even for months. Bacterial infections usually respond well to eye drops containing antibiotics.

Perennial allergic conjunctivitis

People with this condition experience a similar spectrum of symptoms to those with the seasonal form. Symptoms tend to occur year round but are usually milder than the seasonal variety. Most people with perennial allergic conjunctivitis suffer from seasonal exacerbations and may also have other atopic conditions, such as asthma. In severe forms, perennial allergic conjunctivitis can scar the cornea (the thin layer of cells over the eye). This can affect vision.

Atopic keratoconjunctivitis

This is more serious than the seasonal and perennial forms. This condition almost always arises in adults, when atopic dermatitis (see Chapter 8) affects the eye. The affected eye itches intensely and produces large amounts of stringy mucus. People with atopic keratoconjunctivitis might also find light uncomfortable (a symptom called photophobia). Some also find that their vision blurs. The eyelid and skin around the eye often shows crusting and scaling.

Untreated atopic keratoconjunctivitis can lead to a number of complications, including cataracts (where the lens becomes opaque) and damage to the cornea. If you think you have atopic keratoconjunctivitis you should consult your doctor or optician immediately.

Vernal keratoconjunctivitis

This is extremely itchy and sometimes painful. It is also, fortunately, rare. The affected eye may produce a considerable amount of tears. People with vernal keratoconjunctivitis may experience photophobia (aversion to light), feel as if they have a foreign body in their eye, or report blurred vision. Children often rub their eye vigorously.

Vernal keratoconjunctivitis usually appears in children aged between 11 and 13 years. It's rare among people over 30 years of age. Furthermore, the condition tends to be most common in hot, dry climates, and symptoms usually peak in the spring and autumn. Again, if you think you or your child has vernal keratoconjunctivitis you should see your doctor or optician.

Treatment of allergic conjunctivitis

Treatment of atopic and vernal keratoconjunctivitis (see opposite) is best left to specialists. However, management is, broadly, the same as for the allergic forms. In this section we'll look at some treatments for seasonal and perennial allergic conjunctivitis. Many of these are now available from pharmacists; others can be obtained on prescription.

Despite their effectiveness in other allergies, **steroids** are not widely used in the treatment of eye inflammation. Steroid eye drops can cause serious side-effects, such as increasing the risk of infection, glaucoma and cataracts, as well as delaying wound healing. Only specialists should prescribe steroid eye drops.

Many people suffering from allergic rhinoconjunctivitis (conjunctivitis with associated nasal symptoms) find that oral **antihistamines** and other hay fever remedies bought from their local chemist alleviate the eye – as well as the nasal – symptoms. However, nasal sprays, because their effect is largely confined to the nose, may be less effective against conjunctivitis than nasal symptoms.

In mild cases, antihistamine and **vasoconstrictor** eye drops, some of which you can buy over the counter, might relieve the symptoms. Antihistamines block the action of histamine, a major inflammatory mediator (see Chapter 1). Vasoconstrictors close the blood vessels in the eye, so limiting the circulation of white blood cells to the area. (The vasoconstrictors' short duration of action means that the reduction in blood flow doesn't cause damage.)

However, some people with allergic rhinoconjunctivitis find that these over-the-counter medicines do not always work. Fortunately, your GP can offer a number of more effective eye drops for allergic conjunctivitis, such as the following. Each of these has benefits and disadvantages, which you should discuss with your doctor.

- Antihistamines – such as antazoline (combined with a vasoconstrictor such as Otrivine-Antistin), azelastine (Optilast) and emedastine (Emadine) – work rapidly. But antihistamines relieve symptoms for only two to four hours. Because the predominant effect of histamine in the conjunctiva is itching and lacrimation (increased tear production), antihistamines are especially effective against these symptoms. But they tend to be less useful against other symptoms of allergic conjunctivitis – such as redness, oedema (swelling) and mucous discharge – which are produced by other inflammatory mediators. (Azelastine, however, may block inflammatory mediators other than histamine – see below.) Nevertheless, antihistamine eye drops are at least as effective as tablet formulations against these symptoms.[6]

- Nedocromil (Rapitil), sodium cromoglycate (sometimes spelled cromoglicate and available as, for example, Hay-Crom, Opticrom and Vividrin) and lodoxamide (Alomide) are 'mast cell stabilisers' – in other words, they prevent mast cells (see Chapter 1) from producing and releasing their inflammatory mediators. These drugs don't, however, alleviate symptoms: by then the mediators are already released. So this medication is most effective when used to prevent symptoms. This means starting treatment a couple of weeks before the allergy season begins. Treatment needs to continue throughout your allergy season.

There are also a number of other drugs available to treat allergic conjunctivitis, such as the anti-inflammatory ketotifen (Zaditen). Ask your GP or pharmacist for further details.

A considerable body of evidence demonstrates the effectiveness of the above drugs in alleviating the symptoms of allergic conjunctivitis. The following are three examples.

- In one study,[7] 24 golfers allergic to pollen were treated with nedocromil sodium eye drops twice daily for four days before they played a round of golf. The golfers applied an extra dose 15 minutes before they started the game. Symptom severity began to decline around 30 minutes after application, and the improvement lasted for eight to twelve hours. Ninety-two per cent of those participating in the study regarded nedocromil as either moderately or completely effective.
- Other research[8] found that a week's treatment with eye drops containing the antihistamine azelastine markedly improved itching and conjunctival redness in 55 per cent of users after a week. This compared to 14 per cent in the group that received placebo (an inactive but otherwise identical formulation). After 42 days' treatment, 47 per cent of the users reported that

azelastine resolved their symptoms. This compared to 10 per cent in the placebo group. (The placebo might not be entirely inactive – it could wash allergens from the eye.) As mentioned above, azelastine seems to block other inflammatory mediators as well as histamine. This might explain why symptoms continue to improve during prolonged use.

• A third study[9] found that symptoms improved in 53 per cent of people with allergic conjunctivitis when they used ketotifen eye drops twice daily for seven days. Seventy-six per cent reported an improvement after 14 days' treatment. Burning, watery discharge and swelling all improved.

In general, few people develop side-effects to the eye drops used to treat allergic conjunctivitis. Any of the drops discussed above can cause burning, stinging or itching in some people, but such effects tend to be mild and transitory. Some eye drops – such as azelastine and nedocromil – can have a bitter or unusual taste (they can run into the mouth from the eye).

Other drugs can cause specific side-effects. Levocabastine (Livostin) can cause blurred vision and headaches, for example. So it is important to ask your GP about the potential adverse effects and to read the product insert. (See 'Twelve questions to ask your doctor about your drugs', page 105)

Self-help steps

There are a few things you can do to alleviate the symptoms of allergic conjunctivitis. Needless to say, try to avoid the offending allergen by following the tips in Chapter 2. You could also try cold compresses – try soaking a hand flannel in cold water – to relieve the itching. Artificial tears, available from your pharmacist, might also help – these dilute the allergens and counter the effect of antihistamines, which can reduce tear production.

There seems to be no truth to the old wives' tale that regularly eating honey alleviates allergic rhinoconjunctivitis. Researchers compared the effectiveness of two types of honey with corn syrup mixed with synthetic honey flavouring. The subjects of the study didn't know which they received. Honey was no more effective against the symptoms of rhinoconjunctivitis than the corn syrup.[10]

Chapter summary

Conjunctivitis is an inflammation of the thin layer of cells that covers the whites of the eyes and the insides of the eyelids. It is caused by number of allergic and other triggers: for example, almost all hay fever sufferers experience some eye symptoms. Several other eye diseases can cause similar symptoms, so it is important to consult your doctor or optician to make sure that the problem really is allergic conjunctivitis. In most cases, combining eye drops with some simple lifestyle measures alleviates the symptoms.

Chapter 11

Food allergy and intolerance

Few diseases are as controversial as food allergies. Many more people believe that they or their child suffers from food allergies than show an IgE-mediated reaction (see Chapter 1). Despite this, and although until a decade or so ago food allergies were relatively rare, today they are increasingly common. The number of cases – especially in allergy to peanuts and tree nuts – rose sharply during the 1990s.

Several studies highlight the burden imposed by food allergies across much of the industrialised world. A *Health Which?* article in 1997[1] commented that the Ministry of Agriculture, Fisheries and Food (MAFF) learnt of six deaths from nut allergies in the previous year. According to the article, around one in 200 UK children may be allergic to peanuts, while one in 2,000 could be allergic to sesame seeds. These figures suggest that some 300,000 children in the UK may be allergic to peanuts. Indeed, according to other research, between 4 and 8 per cent of children and 1 to 2 per cent of adults are allergic to at least one food.[2]

Food allergies tend to develop during the first couple of years of life,[3] so looking at children offers a good way to assess the scale of the problem. In one study[4] of a group of UK children born in 1989, 0.5 per cent exhibited peanut allergy by four years of age. In a further study[5] of another group of children from the same area, born between 1994 and 1996, 1 per cent had peanut allergies.

The allergic symptoms triggered by foods range from mild irritation around the mouth to rashes, vomiting and diarrhoea. Occasionally, a person may suffer anaphylaxis (see Chapter 4) after ingesting a food. But, although tragic cases where a person dies after eating a peanut can capture the headlines, food-related anaphylaxis is rare.

But not all symptoms that arise after eating certain foods are caused by allergies. For example, about 1 per cent of people in Western countries develop coeliac disease (see box on page 180). And certain foods can exacerbate or trigger other diseases, such as asthma, migraine or irritable bowel syndrome. So, just what do we mean by food allergies? How do they differ from food intolerances?

What are food allergies?

Differentiating food allergy and intolerance can, in some cases, be difficult even for experienced clinicians. Even researchers can't quite agree on a precise definition of food allergy. But in essence – as you'll remember from Chapter 1 – food allergies involve the immune system. In many cases, specific IgE – the allergy antibody – triggers the release of mediators from mast cells when the allergic person comes into contact with specific foods. This sets off the 'immune cascade' outlined in Chapter 1.

However, a number of other non-IgE immune reactions to food can also trigger allergic symptoms, such as constipation, rash, headache and sleeplessness. For example, although up to 40 per cent of children suffering from moderate to severe eczema show evidence of food allergies, not all of these cases of food-exacerbated eczema seem to be mediated by IgE. Unfortunately, researchers do not yet fully understand the mechanisms underlying these non-IgE pathways.

Peanuts – which are not really nuts but are related to legumes (such as peas and beans) – are the best-known food allergen. But almost any food can trigger an allergy in susceptible people. Nevertheless, eggs, milk, peanuts, tree nuts (for example, Brazils), fish, shellfish, soya, wheat, fruits and some vegetables – such as carrots, potatoes and celery – tend to account for most food allergies.

Some people suffer from the food allergy for their entire lives; others seem to grow out of it. For example, around 90 per cent of children allergic to eggs and milk stop experiencing symptoms usually by the age of five years, a report in 2003 by the Royal College of Physicians[6] remarks. Another researcher adds, however, that the time taken for milk allergy to wane can vary from a few months to eight or ten years. In contrast, only a few children seem to lose their allergies to peanuts and tree nuts.

To complicate matters further, cooking can affect the structure of potentially allergenic proteins, such as those in egg whites. So some people allergic to raw eggs can eat them if they are cooked. Nevertheless, people with egg allergies are usually advised to avoid eggs in any form. (This means that they need to steer clear of cakes, biscuits, batters, waffles, pancakes, ice cream, mayonnaise and so on.)[7]

Some people are extremely sensitive to food triggers. Eating 'substantially less' than a single peanut can trigger allergic reactions in susceptible people.[2] Indeed, in highly sensitive people, 100 μg (one ten-thousandth of a gram) of peanut is enough for them to feel a change. Visible signs, such as a rash, can emerge with just 2mg (two-thousandths of a gram). So sometimes peanut residues left on a pan used to cook, for example, a take away stir-fry can trigger symptoms, even if the meal itself doesn't contain peanuts.

Indeed, some allergic people do not even have to eat the food to develop a reaction – people allergic to raw potatoes can experience rhinitis and asthma attacks when peeling spuds, for example. Others have asthma attacks after handling green beans or raw rice. There are even reports of people developing allergic reactions when many packets of roasted peanuts are opened simultaneously during a flight – the peanut dust released into the air triggers the attack.

Inhaled exposure to food allergens may not be as unusual as it sounds. Researchers estimate that about 10 per cent of asthma cases in adults are caused by occupational allergens (see Chapter 5). And food allergens carried in the air seem to account for about 10 per cent of cases of occupational asthma. So inhaled food allergens may play 'a major role' in at least 1 per cent of cases of asthma in adults.[8]

The symptoms of food allergies

Food allergies can cause a range of reactions from mild erythema (skin redness) around the lips to anaphylaxis (see Chapter 4). The first reaction could be mild or severe. More specifically, food allergies can cause the following symptoms (some of these are caused by IgE-mediated reactions, others arise from non-IgE mechanisms):

- urticaria (bumps on the skin), atopic dermatitis and other rashes (see Chapter 8)
- angioedema (see Chapter 8)
- itchy skin
- itchiness or tingling in the mouth (see the 'oral-allergy' syndrome, page 59)
- coughing, trouble breathing, wheezing and throat tightness
- rhinitis
- irritability and sleeplessness
- headache and migraine
- joint pains
- diarrhoea, vomiting, colic and other gastrointestinal symptoms
- anaphylaxis (see Chapter 4).

The symptoms of food allergies depend, to a certain extent, on the person's age and the severity of the reaction. For example, in infants with food allergies, gastrointestinal symptoms tend to predominate. Young children, in particular, may vomit when they ingest the allergen. As children get older, skin, respiratory and other symptoms are more common. But even in adults, the allergic inflammation is most likely to arise in the gut. Skin reactions are the next most common symptoms and, because they are easily seen, may be the most obvious sign. Allergic symptoms usually emerge within ten minutes, but in a few cases may be delayed by up to two hours of eating the food. Severe reactions, including anaphylaxis, tend to emerge and progress rapidly.

Many people with food allergies develop respiratory symptoms, such as a feeling that their throat is closing up or mild asthma. Respiratory symptoms often become especially over-whelming in severe allergic reactions. Against this background, researchers have found that food allergy is a significant risk factor for life-threatening asthma attacks in children. In one study,[9] being admitted to hospital or visiting the Accident and Emergency unit frequently for the condition, which indicates poor control of asthma, was linked to roughly a tenfold increase in the risk of suffering life-threatening asthma. But food allergies increased the likelihood of developing life-threatening asthma almost sixfold. Indeed, half the cases with life-threatening asthma showed food allergy, compared with 10 per cent of controls.

Children with atopic dermatitis and asthma are especially prone to developing respiratory symptoms associated with food allergy. And food allergies often overlap with other common atopic diseases – up to 40 per cent of children with moderate to severe eczema show evidence of food allergies, for example. One study[10] found that 96 per cent of around 560 people with a nut allergy also had another atopic disease. Sixty-three per cent had allergic asthma, 64 per cent had allergic rhinitis and 61 per cent had atopic dermatitis. (Obviously, the subjects commonly had more than one allergic disease.) Many of these people were also allergic to foods other than nuts. Clearly, it is important to determine whether food allergies contribute to a person's poorly controlled asthma, hay fever and eczema.

Food allergy is the most common cause of childhood anaphylaxis (see Chapter 4). And peanuts are the most common cause of these life-threatening allergic reactions. But peanuts aren't the only food that can cause severe allergic reactions – tree nuts, fish and shellfish are also commonly linked to anaphylaxis.[2]

In most cases of fatal food-related anaphylaxis, people knew they had a food allergy, but they were unable to obtain medical advice or took their adrenaline injection too late. The Royal College of Physicians report[6] mentioned earlier notes that most people who use their adrenaline injection within 30 minutes of ingesting the allergen survive. This underscores the importance of ensuring that people at risk of anaphylaxis, as well as parents and carers, are fully aware of the need for emergency treatment and how to administer therapy. As explained in Chapter 4, self-management plans can reduce both the number and severity of anaphylactic reactions.

Coeliac disease

Coeliac disease arises in genetically susceptible people who generate a specific immune response to allergens present in wheat gluten.[11] (Gluten, a mixture of two proteins, gives dough its elasticity.) This immune response is not, however, mediated by IgE (see Chapter 1) and is not strictly speaking an allergy. So gastroenterologists, rather than allergists, manage people with coeliac disease. People with coeliac disease cannot effectively absorb nutrients in their food.

Typically, coeliac disease emerges in young children, when they start eating cereal crops, such as wheat, rye and barley. However, coeliac disease can also occur in adults. So doctors should consider it a possibility in any adult who develops anaemia. People with coeliac disease – especially children – show a range of symptoms, which may include poor growth (failure to thrive), general malnutrition, delayed puberty, chronic diarrhoea, abdominal distension and pain, muscle wasting, poor appetite and behavioural problems. Researchers note that many of the symptoms, such as anaemia, weight loss and bone pain, arise from poor nutrition.[12]

Furthermore, coeliac disease seems to increase the risk of developing gastrointestinal cancer or lymphoma (malignancies of the lymph nodes). Indeed, coeliac disease inevitably damages the gastrointestinal tract. But the various manifestations of coeliac disease and the wide range of associated conditions can make diagnosis difficult.[12]

A strict gluten-free diet – which means avoiding wheat, rye and barley – is the mainstay of management for coeliac disease. Following a gluten-free diet rapidly alleviates symptoms and, after a few months, allows the gastrointestinal damage to heal.[13] However, many people with coeliac disease find following a strict gluten-free diet extremely difficult. Furthermore, commercial foods can be contaminated with traces of gluten. Further advice is available from Coeliac UK.*

What is food intolerance?

People with food intolerance do not experience symptoms as a result of producing specific IgE (see Chapter 1) to a food allergen or by other allergic mechanisms. Despite this, they can suffer some unpleasant symptoms that may, in some cases, mimic those of an allergic reaction. Food intolerance, however, results from a number of non-allergic causes.

Some people, for example, lack an enzyme that digests certain foods. So, for example, some people cannot digest lactose – the sugar in milk. And this can cause gastrointestinal discomfort. In other types of food intolerance, a substance in the food can irritate the gut lining, trigger asthma or produce a number of other symptoms.

For example, some foods contain histamine, one of the key inflammatory mediators released by mast cells (see Chapter 1). In sensitive people, the histamine in wine can trigger sneezing, flushing, headache, itching, breathlessness and urticaria ('hives') – sometimes after a single glass. Indeed, the symptoms can be exactly the same as in the IgE-mediated allergy – after all, histamine is one of the main atopic mediators. Some other foods and drinks, including cheese, fish, sausages, and beer, also contain histamine. The histamine in certain foods might be one reason why some people find that these foods give them a headache or trigger a migraine. Furthermore, bacteria can cause some foods – particular tuna and mackerel – to spoil, which releases high levels of histamine. (In such cases, everyone who eats the fish – not only those who have an allergy – will experience a reaction.)

To complicate matters further, a number of other conditions can be exacerbated by certain foods. For example, milk, wheat and eggs may exacerbate irritable bowel syndrome (IBS). IBS is not really a disease. It's more a collection of symptoms that includes abdominal pain, changes in bowel habit, dyspepsia, passing mucus with stools, and so on. Broadly, however, IBS can be characterised in one of two forms, depending on whether constipation or diarrhoea is the predominant symptom. Up to 70 per cent of people with IBS find that a simple diet of fish and meat with vegetables alleviates symptoms. But you shouldn't cut milk, wheat and eggs from your diet without the support of a dietician. (Your GP can refer you.)

Similarly, some migraine sufferers react to tyramine, an amino acid (one of the building blocks of protein). Cheese, red wine, beer, chocolate and beef are among the common foods and drinks that are especially high in tyramine. A combination of certain foods, along with other triggers (such as stress or lack of sleep), seems to cause the blood vessels supplying the brain to swell. This causes some of the symptoms of migraine. (For more detailed advice on tackling IBS and migraine see *The Which? Guide to Managing Stress*.)

The symptoms of food intolerance

Food intolerance can cause a variety of symptoms, depending on the food. For example, milk intolerance can cause gastrointestinal symptoms, such as bloating and flatulence. Tartrazine, a yellow food dye, can cause asthma and, in some cases, urticaria.

The symptoms of intolerance tend to emerge at least an hour after eating the food. This differs from the typical timescale for allergic reactions to foods (see earlier), which generally emerge more rapidly. This pattern may help distinguish food allergies from intolerance. But, unfortunately, it's not a hard-and-fast rule. The best way to differentiate food allergy from intolerance is to undergo an exclusion diet (see later in this chapter) to identify the 'culprit' food and then have other tests, such as the skin prick test (see Chapter 3), to determine whether an allergic reaction may be responsible.

Managing food allergies

Unfortunately, apart from avoiding the culprit, ensuring that you know the warning signs and knowing how to deal with severe reactions, there is relatively little you can do to manage food allergies. In some cases, doctors may prescribe sodium cromoglycate – a mast cell stabiliser (see Chapter 1) also used in the treatment of asthma, allergic conjunctivitis and rhinitis – in addition to excluding the trigger. However, this needs to be taken before the meal that may contain the allergen. But strict avoidance of the food is really the only effective approach. Obviously, this means you first have to identify the culprit.

Diagnosing food allergies

Unfortunately, when a patient presents to a doctor with symptoms that suggest he or she may have food allergy or intolerance, there are few reliable and easy-to-use tests that allow doctors to confirm the diagnosis.

As a result, a diagnostic industry has emerged, offering a variety of complementary techniques that purport to determine the cause of these allergies. As explained in Chapter 13, there is little, if any, scientific evidence supporting these methods. Researchers comment that many of the complementary diagnostic and therapeutic approaches to food allergy and intolerance are supported by testimonials rather than hard scientific evidence. So the placebo effect (see box on page 200) might be responsible for any benefits that emerge.[14] Moreover, following any advice to exclude foods from your diet could, unless it's under the supervision of a dietician, lead to health problems. If you still feel that you want to explore these approaches you should be very cautious.

Fortunately, however, despite the lack of a single, infallible test, several of the diagnostic tests outlined in Chapter 3, including skin prick tests and laboratory approaches, can help diagnose food allergies.

As mentioned in Chapter 3, however, just because you react on skin prick testing does not necessarily mean that it triggers your asthma, eczema or other allergic symptoms. Indeed, up to half of all positive reactions to foods on skin prick tests are false when investigated on challenge testing. ('Challenge testing' here refers to the reintroduction of the food after it has been excluded from the diet. We discussed this in Chapter 3.)

One study[15] showed that measuring specific IgE (which can be done using laboratory tests – see Chapter 3) identified most children with egg allergy. But the concentration of IgE did not correspond to the dose needed to cause symptoms on challenge testing. Therefore, measuring IgE might not accurately reflect the severity of the allergy. And, because IgE is not responsible for all allergies or any case of intolerance, measuring levels of this antibody doesn't help diagnose these other mechanisms.

For these reasons, food allergies and intolerance are generally diagnosed using exclusion and challenge tests. We looked at these in more detail in Chapter 3, but they can be summarised as follows.

- In a formal exclusion diet, you exclude suspect foods from your diet for five to eight weeks. One of the suspect foods is then reintroduced – the challenge – and you note the severity and frequency of any symptoms in a diary. This is then repeated for the other suspected foods.

- In a less formal exclusion diet, you ban a suspect food from your diet, and record your symptoms before and during the exclusion period. If the symptoms abate, the food might be responsible for your symptoms. About ten days' exclusion should usually be enough to pinpoint the 'culprit' food. If the suspicions are wrong, however, finding the culprit can take months.

- In another variant of the exclusion diet, you exclude everything from your diet apart from a few bland foods. Then you gradually reintroduce a normal diet, noting the response as you become reacquainted with various foods.

Exclusion and other diets should be performed only under the supervision of a qualified dietician. If you try to 'do it yourself', it is very easy to exclude important nutrients in your diet. To avoid nutritional deficiencies – or even overt malnutrition – during the exclusion period, you need to eat alternative foods and be carefully monitored.

There's another good reason why you should diagnose and manage food allergies only under medical supervision. As we have seen, food allergies often overlap with other atopic diseases, which complicates diagnosis and management. For example, a study[16] of adults allergic to at least one fruit found that 65 per cent were allergic to pollen, which caused hay fever, asthma or both. Twenty-eight per cent were allergic to latex. Such 'cross-reactions' between allergens are not uncommon – for more details see Chapter 2.

What about additives, preservatives and dyes?

Many parents worry that artificial additives, preservatives and dyes can cause health problems in their children. In reality, the risk is low. About one in 100 children and one in 500 adults develop reactions to food dyes. The Royal College of Physicians report[6] remarks that food dyes and additives 'only occasionally cause urticaria'. The report also comments that there is no convincing proof that food additives or salicylates (see below) are associated with attention deficit hyperactivity disorder. This is a controversial area and there is clearly a need for further research.

Nevertheless, there is no doubt that some people with asthma are sensitive to the various metabisulphite additives (E220–227). Metabisulphite is a preservative used in dried fruits, pickles, sausages, fruit and on certain vegetables. In these people, metabisulphite can trigger an asthma attack, possibly because the gas sulphur dioxide is released from the food. As we saw in Chapter 2, this pollutant constricts the airways.

In addition, people with aspirin-induced asthma may cross-react to the dye tartrazine (E102), which is used to colour foods and some medicines yellow or orange.

Finally, as we saw in Chapter 5, a group of chemicals known as salicylates, which include aspirin and the other non-steroidal anti-inflammatory drugs (such as ibuprofen), can trigger asthma or rhinitis in sensitive people. Salicylates are also used as food preservatives and occur naturally in certain foods, so may be present in a range of foods from some soft drinks, hot dogs or ice cream to some fruits and vegetables. It is almost impossible to totally avoid salicylate-containing foods, but you can watch out for and steer clear of those foods that seem to particularly exacerbate your symptoms. Keeping a symptom diary (see Chapter 3) may help.

Avoiding food triggers

To avoid the symptoms of food allergies and intolerance you need to avoid the cause. We have seen that, with one exception, there are no effective drug treatments for food allergies – although several approaches are being studied in clinical trials and laboratories. However, it will be years before these are widely used in medical practice.

If someone in your family has a food allergy, shopping can become a difficult, time-consuming task, and eating out can cause particular problems. You need to insist that restaurant staff, including those in take-away establishments, offer detailed information. It might be worth phoning a restaurant in advance. Allergy UK★ offers further support and advice about living with allergies. Suggestions for further reading are given at the back of this book.

When buying food, it is important to read labels carefully, but remember that some allergic trigger foods may be present in minuscule quantities, and not identified. The *Health Which?* article[1] mentioned earlier noted that many foods contain sesame seeds, and these include vegetarian dishes, burger buns, hummous, herbal drinks and bread. But, the article warned, this might not be obvious from the packaging. In June 2002, Allergy UK* introduced a logo that shows a food is free from a particular ingredient that could cause an allergic reaction – for example, wheat-free bread. (Apart from triggering coeliac disease – see page 180 – wheat can also cause allergic reactions in some people.) The logo does not, however, cover nut-free products.

Sometimes food packaging may describe peanuts as 'groundnuts' or 'arachis' – so be careful. Some skin ointments, cosmetics and toiletries contain arachis oil, so make sure you read the list of ingredients. Furthermore, some foods – such as sweets, loaves bought from a baker or sandwiches – may be unlabelled. And even so-called vegetable oil may contain nuts. On the other hand, the risk of contamination during manufacture means that many products are labelled 'may contain nuts' when they do not. But don't take the risk.

Genetic modification of food adds a further complication. As noted in a *Health Which?* article in June 2002,[17] genetically modified (GM) food could, in theory at least, reduce the risk of severe allergies by removing from common food triggers, such as peanuts, the protein that triggers the allergy. On the other hand, GM can also add allergens. In one case, a company added proteins from Brazil nuts to soya to increase the nutritional quality. Research on the modified soya stopped after scientists realised that the product could trigger allergies in people allergic to Brazil nuts. Supporters of GM suggest that the regulatory process should mean that the risk of allergic reactions is low. However, the article pointed out that there is also a possibility that new allergies could emerge in genetically modified foods.

If you think this sounds as though nobody is sure just what genetic modification means for people with food allergies, you are right! Until the issue is resolved, it's best to play safe, read the labels carefully and keep informed about the developments in this controversial area. By law, foods must be labelled as genetically modified if they contain more than 1 per cent GM produce. Several groups, including Consumers' Association (CA), want all ingredients derived from genetically modified sources to be listed on the label. If you support this, you could try writing to your MP and MEP. See www.which.co.uk for more information about CA's campaign in this area.

If your child has a food allergy, it's important to warn teachers, babysitters and other carers about the risk. This is particularly important if the child is at risk of anaphylaxis – when the adult responsible should also know how to administer the adrenaline injections. This is covered in more detail in Chapter 4.

It's also worth discouraging your child from sharing food at school or at parties. You might want to supply packed lunches and food to take to a party. Living with a food allergy – or a child who has a food allergy – is difficult. But following the steps outlined in this chapter can help people with these allergies lead as normal lives as possible.

Chapter summary

Food allergies are increasingly common, although many more people believe that they have the condition than actually do. Many of these other people suffer from unpleasant food intolerances. The most effective way to identify food allergies and intolerance is by exclusion and challenge diets. To distinguish allergy from intolerance it may be necessary to undergo some of the tests described in Chapter 3. Unfortunately, apart from avoiding the culprit, there is relatively little you can do to manage food allergies.

Chapter 12

Drug-induced allergies

In 1981, more than 20,000 people in Spain developed breath-lessness, joint pains, fevers, rashes and numerous other unpleasant symptoms. Several hundred died. Researchers eventually discovered the cause: rapeseed oil that had been illegally adulterated with a toxic chemical called aniline. The exact mechanism under-lying the reactions remains something of a mystery. It's clear, however, that this so-called 'toxic oil syndrome' was caused at least in part by the immune system.

The toxic oil syndrome offers a striking reminder that chemicals in the environment can promote serious, even fatal, immune-based reactions. Fortunately, such public health disasters are rare. But, on the other hand, most drugs are chemicals – and these too can trigger a variety of immune-based reactions.

Adverse drug reactions – the correct term for 'side-effects' – range from the predictable to the rare and idiosyncratic. This chapter reviews one type of adverse drug reaction: allergic and hypersensitivity reactions. Between 75 and 80 per cent of adverse drug reactions (for example, a dry mouth associated with anti-histamines or thrush during antibiotic treatment) arise from the drug's pharmacology – that is, its characteristic biological actions. Another 5 to 10 per cent of adverse reactions are caused by one of several immune mechanisms: these are the allergic and hypersensi-tivity reactions. Those caused by IgE (see Chapter 1) are known as drug allergies. Hypersensitivity reactions arise from several other immune mechanisms. The remaining 10 to 20 per cent of adverse drug reactions are 'unpredictable' and arise through non-immune pathways.[1]

In this chapter we'll take a brief look at drug-induced allergic and hypersensitivity reactions. In particular, we will focus on penicillin, which is the most common cause of drug-induced allergies. The general principles exemplified by penicillin apply to many other drugs.

If, after starting a new drug, you feel anything unexpected – for example, if you find that you have difficulty breathing, feel faint or develop a skin rash – talk to your pharmacist or GP. If you show symptoms of anaphylaxis (see Chapter 4), seek medical attention immediately. Remember that, as you take drugs for several days, the re-exposure can rapidly follow the initial sensitisation (that is, the tendency to develop allergic symptoms the next time you are exposed) – which may be within the same course of treatment.

How common are adverse reactions to drugs?

Pharmacologists – scientists who study a drug's biological actions – have long sought to find a 'magic bullet' for each disease: a drug that specifically targets the affected cells without causing adverse reactions. They're still looking. Every drug currently on the market causes at least some side-effects in some people. Indeed, researchers have commented that 'adverse reactions to drugs are very common in everyday medical practice'.[2] Nevertheless, as biologists understand more about the molecular basis of disease, drugs are increasingly accurately targeted. This means that pharmacologists are better able to differentiate the therapeutic effects from those that cause adverse reactions.

Overall, between 5 and 15 per cent of prescriptions lead to adverse drug reactions.[1] (The chance of developing adverse drug reactions depends on several factors, including your genetic make-up, the drug, the dose and the formulation.) The vast majority of these adverse reactions are mild and transitory. Only very rarely are they fatal.

Antibiotics and non-steroidal anti-inflammatory drugs (NSAIDs) seem to be the drugs most likely to be associated with adverse drug reactions, largely because they are prescribed very commonly. For example, as we saw in Chapter 5, aspirin and NSAIDs can exacerbate asthma and rhinitis. NSAIDs can, in addition, cause a wide range of other side-effects, including bleeding from, and ulcers in, the gastrointestinal tract; nausea and vomiting; and headaches and dizziness.

While 5 to 15 per cent may not seem to be an especially high proportion, doctors prescribe a staggering amount of drugs. As a result, a lot of people develop adverse drug reactions. The Association of the British Pharmaceutical Industry estimates that in 2000, for example, community pharmacists (those in the high street, supermarket or a GP's surgery rather than hospitals) dispensed some 637.5 million prescriptions – that's almost 11 prescriptions for every person in the UK.

How common are drug-induced allergies?

As mentioned earlier, 5 to 10 per cent of adverse drug reactions are caused by immune mechanisms.[1] Furthermore, although estimates vary, between 1 and 10 per cent of the UK population is allergic to penicillin – the classic example of a drug-induced allergy, which we'll consider in detail later.

But it is difficult to gain an accurate measure of the scale of the problem posed by allergic and hypersensitivity reactions. As a report in 2003 from the Royal College of Physicians[3] remarks, under-reporting of drug allergy is rife. The report notes that few hospitals have the facilities to fully investigate suspected cases of drug allergy and that there are few reliable, objective diagnostic tests. Moreover, diagnosing drug allergy and hypersensitivity can be difficult. Skin hypersensitivity reactions can mimic several skin diseases, including cancer, bacterial infection and psoriasis (a skin disease in which an aberrant immune system leads to silvery scales on the skin. It seems to arise from a predominance of Th_1-cells – see Chapter 1).[4]

Nevertheless, we can arrive at an approximation of the incidence of serious allergic reactions. The Royal Collge of Physicians report[3] notes that a study from the Netherlands found 40 to 50 cases of drug-induced anaphylaxis each year between 1974 and 1994, from a population of 15 million. A total of 21 people died as a result – roughly one a year – from drug-induced anaphylaxis.

It is important, however, to keep the risks of developing a drug-induced allergy in perspective. Only about one in 15,000 people taking a drug develops a life-threatening anaphylactic reaction. Moreover, perhaps three times as many people believe themselves to be allergic to a drug than show reactions on diagnostic tests, such as skin prick tests or a challenge test (see Chapter 3). Many of these people may have, in the past, suffered a pharmacological side-effect that they misattribute to allergies.

Avoiding allergic and hypersensitivity reactions

If you have suffered an allergic reaction to a drug, you should keep a written record of this on yourself at all times. This helps your GP, or a doctor in an Accident and Emergency department, when he or she needs to prescribe a drug. You should always let any healthcare professional, including dentists and pharmacists, know that you have suffered a suspected or confirmed allergic reaction in the past – in many cases, doctors cannot easily access your entire medical history.

The symptoms of allergic and hypersensitivity reactions

Drug-induced allergies can cause symptoms on almost any part of the body. Nevertheless, urticaria and other skin reactions (see Chapter 8) and conjunctivitis (see Chapter 10) are common. Furthermore, topical medications – those that are applied to the outside of the body – can cause contact dermatitis.[1,5]

The most common drug-related skin reaction is a morbilliform rash: a red, spotty rash that appears within one and three weeks of the start of treatment. The rash begins on the trunk and spreads to the limbs. Morbilliform rashes seem to arise from the activation of T-cells, a type of white blood cell, specific to that drug. These T-cells release inflammatory mediators (see Chapter 1 for more about this process) that trigger skin inflammation, which leads to the rash.

In most cases, the skin rashes are unsightly rather than life threatening. But two reactions – Stevens-Johnson syndrome and toxic epidermal necrolysis – appear as blisters on the skin and the mucous membranes, such as inside the mouth. Such symptoms indicate the need for prompt treatment: the condition can be serious and even fatal.[1]

Why do we mount an allergic reaction to some drugs?

Researchers are beginning to understand why some people develop an allergic – (i.e. IgE-based) reaction to a drug while others do not.

For example, people with atopy (a genetic tendency to develop IgE in response to allergic triggers) may be more likely to develop serious reactions, including anaphylaxis (see Chapter 4).

Furthermore, genetically determined differences in the way that the body metabolises and excretes drugs (see box below) can influence the risk of developing an adverse drug reaction. For example, researchers have identified a gene linked to an increased risk of insulin allergy.

Metabolic pathways

When we say that the body metabolises a drug, we mean that the body breaks the chemical down – usually, but not always, into less toxic forms. These 'break-down products' – called metabolites – are then excreted, often in the urine, faeces or both. As you get older your ability to break drugs down and excrete them may decline. This is one reason why the dose of some drugs given to older people is lower than that prescribed to younger people. Similarly, the doctor may adjust the dose if you have a liver or kidney disease. (You should always let the pharmacist and GP know if you suffer from liver or kidney diseases when you buy prescription drugs or over-the-counter medicines – don't rely on your medical records being up to date.)

A family of enzymes (special proteins in the body that speed up chemical reactions) – known collectively as the cytochrome P450s – is responsible for many critical metabolic reactions. Genetically determined differences in the type and activity of cytochrome P450s can alter the way the body handles drugs. For example, you might metabolise the drug rapidly, in which case the therapeutic effect will quickly wear off. Other people might metabolise it slowly, which may leave them vulnerable to side-effects.

The success of the human genome project and other advances in molecular biology gave researchers considerable insights into the genetic factors that influence metabolic capacity. So in the next few years – it's already a research tool – doctors will be able to 'scan' your genetic profile to determine how likely you are to develop adverse reactions to certain drugs. The technique is currently being assessed in clinical studies.

Only certain drugs trigger IgE-mediated reactions. As noted in Chapter 1, most allergic triggers – allergens – are proteins. This means they are fairly large, at least on a molecular level. So some drugs, such as streptokinase (a clot-buster used in, for example, heart attacks), vaccines and insulin can directly act as allergens.

Most drugs, on the other hand, are relatively small. So small, in fact, that they normally elude the immune system. But certain drugs or their metabolites (break-down products) are especially reactive and can bind to proteins. Researchers describe these drugs and metabolites as 'haptens'.

For example, aniline, the contaminant responsible for the toxic oil syndrome, does not directly trigger an immune reaction. Its metabolites, however, are highly reactive and can act as haptens. Similarly, penicillin triggers allergic reactions by acting as a hapten. The immune system then recognises the combination of the hapten and protein as foreign and mounts an allergic response.

Drug allergies emerge between seven and ten days after the person starts taking the medicine. This reflects the time taken for the body to produce specific IgE (see Chapter 1) for the first time. The body is then primed to respond to the drug when the person is exposed to it a second time – which, as we noted earlier, might be during the same course of treatment.

Not all allergic symptoms arising from taking a drug are atopic (IgE-mediated). Certain drugs – including opioid painkillers, such as morphine, and an antibiotic called vancomycin – can trigger histamine release. This leads to similar symptoms as an IgE-mediated allergic reaction. Because an immune mechanism isn't involved, doctors refer to these cases as 'pseudoallergic' reactions. Moreover, because the body doesn't have to produce IgE, pseudoallergic reactions can occur rapidly.

Penicillin can cause haemolytic anaemia (low levels of red blood cells) when IgG or IgM, two other types of antibody, attack cells coated with the complex of drug plus hapten. Furthermore, drug–antibody complexes can form deposits in tissues and cause inflammation. This can lead to tissue damage, especially in the joints, kidneys and lungs. Such reactions are relatively rare, at least in the drugs prescribed by GPs for common diseases.

Other causes of drug-induced allergies are drugs used during operations – muscle relaxants, opioid painkillers and anaesthetics –

which cause anaphylactic or anaphylactoid reactions (see Chapter 4) in about 1 in 6,000 people who receive general anaesthetics. About 6 per cent of these cases prove fatal. (So the risk of suffering a potentially fatal reaction during general anaesthesia is relatively low – about 1 in 100,000.)

Because the incidence of these types of reactions is fairly low, the following section looks in detail at the most common cause of drug-induced allergies: atopic reactions to penicillin and related drugs. These chemical cousins of penicillin, such as ampicillin (Penbritin), amoxicillin (also spelled amoxycillin, brand name Amoxil), flucloxacillin (Floxapen) and many more – created when chemists made minor variations to the basic chemical structure – are collectively known as penicillins. There are several other groups of antibiotics, with still others in development.

Allergy to penicillin

In 1928, Alexander Fleming made a discovery that changed the world. Fleming was researching a group of bacteria called *Staphylococci*, which cause – among several unpleasant and serious diseases – boils, carbuncles, abscesses, pneumonia and septicaemia (blood poisoning).

Fleming left a Petri dish of *Staphylococci* on his bench while he went on holiday. When he returned, a mould – *Penicillium* – had contaminated the culture, destroying the surrounding *Staphylococci*. Later, researchers discovered that the mould secreted a chemical that destroyed *Staphylococci*. They called the chemical penicillin, and it ultimately led to the development of today's antibiotics.

It's hard to overstate the importance of antibiotics. They've saved countless lives. Diseases once feared by our parents and grandparents – such as tuberculosis, pneumonia and scarlet fever – are now rare, at least in the UK and the rest of the developed world.

Antibiotics only kill or prevent the replication of bacteria. They do not eradicate viral infections (such as flu or the common cold) or parasitic infections – in fact, they should really be called antibacterial drugs. (So don't ask your doctor for antibiotics if your child comes down with a sniffle. This just contributes to resistance – and the emergence of so-called 'super-bugs' that don't respond well to antibiotics. This is an issue we'll return to below.)

Moreover, each antibiotic shows a spectrum of action. The 'broad spectrum' antibiotics attack several types of bacteria; others have a narrower action. Even within a particular class, the antibiotics can show differences in their spectrum of action. Furthermore, the increasing number of resistant strains means that an antibiotic's spectrum of action may be in flux.

Antibiotics' specificity for bacteria means that they tend not to cause side-effects. Nevertheless, between 0.7 to 10 per cent of people taking penicillin develop adverse drug reactions.[6] Antibiotics' side-effects include (depending on the drugs and the dose) diarrhoea, nausea, vomiting, headaches, convulsions and jaundice. But, as one researcher remarks, 'allergic and hypersensitivity responses are the most common, and most misunderstood, adverse reactions to penicillin'.[7]

Estimates of the proportion of the population that is allergic to penicillin vary widely – from 1 to 10 per cent. As we've mentioned, penicillins can cause 'true' (IgE) allergic reactions and hypersensitivity reactions, such as haemolytic anaemia (see page 193). The IgE-mediated effects can cause bronchoconstriction (narrowing of the airways – see Chapter 5), swelling in the larynx (voice box), pruritis (itching), skin rashes and anaphylaxis. Indeed, between 1 and 4 per cent of people taking any penicillin develop a rash.[8]

Moreover, about 1 in 200 people develop anaphylaxis (see Chapter 4) after taking penicillin. The risk of anaphylaxis is highest with penicillin injections, which are usually given in hospital, than with tablets. The reaction is life-threatening in only 1 in 15,000 people. However, because penicillins are among the most widely used drugs, they account for three-quarters of deaths caused by anaphylaxis.[9]

Serious reactions, such as anaphylaxis, tend to emerge within an hour of taking the antibiotic. Indeed, in most cases anaphylaxis develops within 5 to 30 minutes, although the symptoms can occur up to 72 hours after you take the drug.[7] Again, as a general rule, the more rapidly the allergic reaction emerges, the more serious it is. As with any anaphylactic reaction, you should seek immediate medical attention.

Diagnosis and management of adverse drug reactions

Doctors diagnose allergic and hypersensitivity reactions based mainly on clinical signs and symptoms. However, laboratory and other diagnostic tests, described in Chapter 3, can help in some cases. For example, pseudoallergic reactions (see page 193), by triggering mast-cell degranulation (see Chapter 1), produce symptoms clinically identical to IgE-mediated reactions. Because pseudoallergic reactions are not associated with IgE to the drug, the two can be distinguished using, for example, a RAST test (see pages 57–8). Skin prick and patch testing may help identify the cause and may be especially valuable for suspected penicillin allergy (that is, IgE-mediated). However, patch testing for drug allergies is still under investigation. Moreover, false-positives and false-negatives can occur with skin prick tests. Specific tests for IgE against some drugs – including amoxicillin, ampicillin and cefaclor – may be available in regional hospitals. Specialist allergy centres can also offer drug provocation, although these tend to be used only as a last diagnostic resort.[3]

Drug allergies and hypersensitivity reactions are managed by removing the triggering drug and prescribing an alternative. Understandably, doctors and dentists are cautious about offering penicillin to people with a history of allergic reactions to the drug. That's why they'll always ask whether you are allergic to penicillin. However, one researcher remarks that clinicians' fear of triggering anaphylaxis might lead to undue caution.[7] So a doctor might 'over-diagnose penicillin allergy', based on patients simply saying that they previously suffered an allergic reaction, rather than checking by using some of the diagnostic measures. (Partly, this may reflect the fact that they don't have the time or resources to investigate drug allergies.) Moreover, only between 10 and 20 per cent of people who say that they are allergic to penicillin react on skin prick testing.[8] (Of course, you should still tell your doctor if you believe that you have suffered an allergic reaction. But, at least, the figures are reassuring.)

Doctors' caution in prescribing penicillin obviously helps avoid the risk of setting off an allergic reaction. But, on the other hand, over-caution contributes to the spread of bacterial resistance – because doctors may resort to more potent antibiotics than are needed to treat disease. This leads to the development of 'super-bugs', resistant to almost every antibiotic, and many doctors are worried that this might soon mean we don't have any drugs left to treat potentially life-threatening infections. Already doctors are down to the last one or two effective antibiotics for some serious diseases in some hospitals.

Fortunately, there are alternative antibiotics to penicillin that can be prescribed for most common infections. People who are allergic to penicillin are, however, also more likely than the population as a whole to react to another group of antibiotics, called the cephalosporins, which includes cefuroxime (Zinacef, Zinnat), cefamandole (Kefadol), cefprozil (Cefzil) and cefaclor (Distaclor). Around 8 per cent of people allergic to penicillin are also hypersensitive to cephalosporins. In contrast, only 2 per cent of people who do not have a penicillin allergy react to cephalosporins.[7] Nevertheless, there are still alternatives to both penicillins and cephalosporins, although how long this will remain the case, given the rise in antibacterial resistance, isn't clear.

Chapter summary

Adverse reactions to drugs are very common: between 5 and 15 per cent of prescriptions lead to adverse drug reactions. Five to 10 per cent of adverse drug reactions are caused by one of several immune mechanisms: these are the allergic and hypersensitivity reactions. Those caused by IgE are known as drug allergies; hypersensitivity reactions arise from several other immune mechanisms. Most of the allergic and hypersensitivity symptoms caused by drugs are relatively mild – dermatitis, urticaria and conjunctivitis, for example. Only about 1 in 15,000 people taking a drug develops a life-threatening anaphylactic reaction. So it is important to keep the dangers in perspective – for most people, the benefits of drugs far outweigh the risks. However, if you find that you have difficulty breathing, feel faint or develop a skin rash after starting a new drug, talk to your pharmacist or GP. If you show symptoms of anaphylaxis seek medical attention immediately.

Chapter 13

Complementary medicine and allergies

Many people living with the allergies we've discussed in the book turn to complementary and alternative medicine (CAM). Often, complementary and alternative therapies are lumped together. However, 'complementary' tends to refer to those therapies that are used *alongside* conventional medicine and that have a degree of acceptance by mainstream doctors – acupuncture, homeopathy and osteopathy, for example. In contrast, 'alternative' tends to refer to those therapies that are used *instead of* mainstream medicine and that are in general not accepted by most conventional doctors – for example, crystal healing, colour therapy and some diagnostic techniques (see pages 201–3). Some people undoubtedly benefit from alternative therapies, although critics suggest that this is largely due to the placebo effect (see box on page 200). Whether you try complementary or alternative therapy, you should never change or stop your conventional treatments without talking to your doctor. If your symptoms have improved, you should be able to reduce the dose of any medication under medical supervision.

Over the years, a large number of CAMs have been suggested as possible treatments for allergies. There isn't space to cover all of these here. So in this chapter we'll look at the most widely used therapies and, in particular, those that have been subjected to scientific scrutiny. You can find more information about some other techniques used in allergies, for example, autogenic training, nutritional therapy and biofeedback, in *The Which? Guide to Complementary Therapies*.

Several factors seem to drive the increasing interest in complementary and alternative medicine among people with allergies. In some cases, people hope that CAM will reduce the amount of medication they need, especially if they are taking, for example, high-dose oral steroids. There's also an impression (which is not necessarily true) that natural treatments are safer than the products of the pharmaceutical industry. In other cases, using CAM can help people feel more empowered, more actively involved in decision-making about their condition and more in control of their disease.[1] And sometimes people consult CAM therapists because they are dissatisfied with the conventional diagnosis and treatments. For example, they may seek help from a CAM practitioner because conventional doctors do not accept that their symptoms have an allergic basis.[2]

Many people undoubtedly benefit from CAM. Indeed, as we'll see, scientific studies show that some CAMs offer direct therapeutic benefits against a particular allergy. Then there are the psychological benefits that arise from taking control of your problems. Moreover, many CAMs aid relaxation, and this can have a non-specific effect on many diseases. Excessive stress may not *cause* many diseases, but it undoubtedly can exacerbate them. (See *The Which? Guide to Managing Stress* for more on the link between stress and psychological or physical ailments.)

Heightened emotions and stress can, for example, trigger an asthma attack and can exacerbate the symptoms of eczema. And allergies can also cause stress: living with food allergies, for instance, can be very stressful. So it's easy to see why relaxation and some CAMs can help. These benefits can complement – but not replace – conventional approaches to allergy management.

Unfortunately, few CAMs for allergic diseases have been subjected to the same type of rigorous scientific scrutiny that drugs have to undergo to reach the market. For example, including a placebo can prove difficult. And many of the studies that purport to show a benefit are poorly designed. So it's hard to draw any firm general conclusions about the effectiveness of CAM in allergic diseases. Further studies are needed for almost every therapy. But, as researchers point out, a lack of evidence doesn't necessarily mean that the therapy is ineffective.[1] It's possible that the appropriate studies haven't been performed. Despite this, you should be wary of CAM practitioners who point to testimonials only rather than hard scientific data. You should always ask whether formal scientific

The placebo effect

A placebo is an intervention – which includes drugs, surgery or a complementary approach – used to alleviate a symptom, but which is either ineffective or not specifically effective in that condition.[3] The word 'placebo' derives from the Latin for 'I please'.

The mind can exert a powerful influence over the body. So some people feel better when they receive a drug, even if it's not biologically effective. This effect contributes to the therapeutic benefit of many conventional drugs. So, in many studies to prove that a medicine works, some people receive the active drug while another group receives a placebo – one that is exactly the same in appearance, taste and so on, but which lacks the active ingredient. (This is sometimes known, somewhat inaccurately, as a 'sugar pill'.) So for example, in an asthma study one group may receive the active drug, while the other receives an inhaler that doesn't contain the medicine. In an atopic dermatitis study, one group receives a cream containing the active drug; the other receives the cream without the drug – known as the vehicle.

Neither the doctor nor the patient knows which is which. This so-called 'double blind' design attempts to rule out any unintentional bias. Any difference between the benefit produced by the placebo and the active medicine is, therefore, likely to be caused by the drug. Although it is possible to design such studies in, for example, herbal and homeopathic medicines, in many CAMs it is difficult to design a placebo to which both the patient and the therapist are blinded. (The same problem also applies to trials of a number of conventional therapies, such as some surgical procedures.) However, well-controlled studies are available in some areas, as we'll see over the course of this chapter.

studies have been performed and check using a reputable source, such as *The Which? Guide to Complementary Therapies, Which? Medicine* (see Further reading), or the references in the Bibliography.

In some cases, CAMs can cause side-effects. Herbal medicines, for example, are potentially powerful drugs – after all morphine, the most powerful painkiller we have, comes from a plant. Several cancer drugs are derived directly or indirectly from plants. Even aspirin is a chemical modification of a plant chemical long-used in herbal medicine. And, herbal remedies can cause a number of side-effects, including allergic contact dermatitis and liver, kidney and heart damage[4] as well as breathing problems.

Furthermore, as we noted in Chapter 11, exclusion and other diets should be performed only under the supervision of a qualified dietician. To avoid nutritional deficiencies, you need to follow a carefully designed dietary plan. So you should think carefully about following any advice on exclusion diets offered on the basis of scientifically unproven complementary diagnostic techniques. Researchers note that there have 'been many false and misleading claims and serious harm may be caused by misdiagnosis or delays in appropriate treatment'.[2]

For all these reasons, when considering any complementary or alternative medicine, it is always worth checking with the appropriate regulatory body that the practitioner who offers the treatment is qualified (where available, details of these bodies are given in the relevant sections of this chapter). Bear in mind also that 'off-the-shelf' treatments are unlikely to be effective for any allergy. The treatment needs to be individually tailored from a qualified practitioner. And you should never stop or change the dose of your conventional medication without speaking to your doctor first.

This chapter considers the scientific basis – if any – for some CAMs for allergic diseases. We'll begin with one of the most controversial areas: alternative diagnostic tests. The therapies are then listed in alphabetical order

Alternative diagnostic tests

Some alternative practitioners offer a number of diagnostic tests that purport to determine the cause of the allergy-related symptoms. For instance:

- **electrodermal testing** (for example, the Vega Test), one of the most commonly used alternative diagnostic tests, claims to link changes in the skin's electrical resistance with allergies. The suspected allergen is placed in a low-voltage electrical circuit in contact with the skin. By measuring changes in electrical resistance, the practitioner claims to be able to identify whether you are allergic to foods and inhaled allergens

- in the **cytotoxic food test** – also called the leuco-cytotoxic test – the practitioner places a drop of blood on a slide coated with a possible food allergen. If, under the microscope, white blood cells seem distorted or swollen, then you're supposed to be allergic to that food
- in **iridology**, the practitioner looks at your iris to determine the colour, texture and location of pigment flecks. Each section of your iris, the theory goes, represents part of your body. Based on the iridology results, practitioners offer treatment using herbs, vitamins and minerals.

But there is no good scientific evidence that any of these alternative diagnostic methods work. Indeed, a report in 2003 by the Royal College of Physicians[5] dismissed the claims made by advocates of these and many other alternative diagnostic methods (see box opposite). The report said there was no validated use for any of these tests. In other words, scientific studies failed to show that the various tests diagnosed allergy.

For example, the Royal College of Physicians noted that hair analysis – which claims to determine your health, nutritional, vitamin and mineral status – is often performed in laboratories that do not use validated methods or standardised materials. In any case, there is no evidence that a low concentration of a particular vitamin or mineral in hair reflects deficiencies in the body's stores. For one thing, dyes and bleaches can influence hair's mineral content. The report also noted that 'a number of controlled trials' suggest that the cytotoxic food test does not effectively diagnose allergies to food or to inhaled allergens.

As we saw in Chapter 3, there is no simple, safe and infallible test for allergy or for a specific allergen. Doctors combine a careful review of your symptoms and your history with, as appropriate, general and specific tests, to gain an insight into the cause of your symptoms and to help devise drug and lifestyle strategies that enable you to live with your allergy. If someone devised a simple and specific test that could be scientifically validated, doctors would probably leap at the chance to use it.

Obviously, the decision to employ one of these tests is yours. But at the very least you should treat any claims and suggestions cautiously. And, again, you should never exclude foods from your or your child's diet based on one of these tests alone: always seek medical advice first.

Diagnostic tests for allergies without a validated use

Adapted from the Royal College of Physicians report[5]

- Electrodermal testing (e.g. Vega Test)
- Hair analysis
- Cytotoxic food test (leuco-cytotoxic test)
- NuTron test (a mechanised system that analyses blood)
- Iridology
- Pulse test (measures increases in pulse after consuming a food)

Active relaxation

Relaxation means more than curling up with a good book or watching your favourite television programme. It is an active process based on the principle that mind and body are linked – you cannot be mentally tense and have a relaxed body, and vice versa – so relaxing the body relaxes the mind. But to relax you have to actively control your body. So this process can be described as 'active relaxation'. Active relaxation may help reduce your risk of having an emotionally triggered allergic exacerbation and increases the likelihood that you will stay calm during an attack of asthma or anaphylaxis.

Overall, however, the evidence that active relaxation benefits asthma is contradictory. For example, one group of researchers reviewed the evidence examining whether active relaxation alleviated asthma.[6] They found that many of the studies were not well designed. On the other hand, designing studies to assess active relaxation isn't easy: how do you include a placebo group (see page 200), for example? Nevertheless, two of five studies assessing active relaxation suggested that they benefited people with asthma. By reducing stress, active relaxation should also help you live with allergic diseases. And you can learn these techniques yourself.

One type of active relaxation – progressive muscular relaxation – aims to relax each part of your body in turn, as follows.

- Lie on the floor with a pillow under your head.
- After a few deep breaths, concentrate on your toes. Then say to yourself: 'My toes are tingling. they are becoming numb ... they are feeling heavier and heavier ... They are feeling increasingly relaxed . . . the tension is draining away.'
- When your toes feel relaxed, move on to your calves. Say to yourself: 'My calves are relaxed ... they are feeling softer and heavier ... they are feeling numb and more relaxed ... the tension is draining away.'
- Once your calves are relaxed, move on to your thighs. Work through the rest of your body in an upward direction (hands, arms, torso, shoulders, face).
- Once you have worked up to your forehead, lie still for a few minutes before standing up.

Using the second approach, called tension-relaxation, you tense a muscle for about ten seconds before relaxing. As with progressive muscular relaxation, the whole body is involved. Each exercise is repeated three times for each part of the body, slowly, gently and gradually. You repeat the set twice, so tensing and relaxing each group of muscles nine times. After this you rest for 20 to 30 minutes. You should master one muscle group at a time, so it could take two or three months before you can tense and relax your whole body.

- Lie on the floor with a pillow under your head, or sit in a chair that supports your back.
- To relax your hands, put them by your sides. Now clench your fists as hard as you can. Hold the fists for ten seconds. Now slowly relax your fists and let your hands hang loosely by your sides.
- When focusing on your shoulders, shrug them as high as possible; when concentrating on the back, arch your back as high as you can, leaving only your head and buttocks touching the chair or floor.
- Tense your muscles when you inhale. During the tension do not hold your breath, but breathe slowly and rhythmically. Then exhale as you relax.

After practising tension-relaxation exercises for a few months, you will come to recognise when your muscles are tense. Most of us live for years with considerable muscle tension, so our bodies become used to a certain level. But this means that we cannot gauge the true state of our muscles. Tension-relaxation exercises familiarise us with our muscles. If you suffer from back problems you should talk to your doctor or physiotherapist before performing tension-relaxation exercises.

The golden rules of relaxation

Whichever technique you choose, following a few simple rules will help you make the most of your relaxation sessions.

- Try to relax every day. The best time is first thing in the morning – the house tends to be quieter and interruptions are less likely.
- Avoid relaxation exercises last thing at night – you will probably not be able to concentrate as well and you could fall asleep rather than relax.
- Do not relax on a full stomach. After a meal, blood diverts from your muscles to your stomach – trying to relax tense muscles on a full stomach can cause cramps. As relaxation exercises increase your awareness of your body's functions, a full stomach can be a distraction.
- Take the phone off the hook or put on the answerphone.
- Play a favourite piece of music, not too loud. Many people find music helps them relax.
- Make yourself comfortable and shut your eyes.
- Concentrate on your breathing. Most of us breathe shallowly, using the upper parts of our lungs. However, to relax you need to breathe deeply and slowly without gasping. Put one hand on your chest and the other on your abdomen. Breathe normally. You may find – especially if you are tense – that the hand on your chest moves, while the hand on the abdomen remains almost still. The hand on your stomach should rise and fall while the one on your chest hardly alters.

Acupuncture

Acupuncture, one of the oldest medical treatments, remains one of the most widely used CAMs. Archaeologists have uncovered stone acupuncture needles dating from 10,000 BC and the first acupuncture texts were written over 2,000 years ago. Today, over three million healers practise acupuncture worldwide, most of these in Asia. Acupuncture's roots lie deep in Eastern philosophy. But Western doctors and CAM practitioners increasingly use acupuncture – although approaches can differ.

The Chinese believe that every organ, process and action of the human body contains 'chi' (also translated as 'qi' or 'ki'), a vital energy. Chi flows throughout the body, but is concentrated in meridians that link the internal organs.

Traditional acupuncturists believe that diseases arise when some-thing – stress, anxiety, fear, grief, infections or trauma, and so on – disturbs the flow or levels of chi. They suggest that too much or too little chi in a particular part of the body can cause disease. For example, hay fever is said to arise partly from a weakness in chi in the nose. Acupuncture aims to balance the flow of chi along these meridians and so prevent and treat illness.

Because chi flows along meridians, acupuncture needles inserted into one part of your body may influence organs some distance away. So to treat asthma, for example, traditional acupuncturists may needle the end of the meridian for the lungs. Alternatively, they may needle two points on the back or a point at the top of the breastbone.

Western medical acupuncturists tend to apply the same tech-niques but, in addition to the traditional acupuncture points, they use so-called 'symptomatic points' to relieve particular symptoms, or 'trigger points'. The latter are unrelated to traditional meridians. When pressed, trigger points evoke a sensation in another part of the body – usually pain or discomfort. Injury, strain, stress, damp, cold, infection or muscle tension can cause trigger points. For example, when we are stressed we tense our muscles. Over time, muscle tension leads to trigger points, which in turn may establish other trigger points.

Conventional doctors use acupuncture to treat a number of condi-tions. According to conventional medical theory, acupuncture works by stimulating the release of natural chemicals, including painkillers in the brain called endorphins. So some physicians use acupuncture on detoxification programmes, to provide pain relief in childbirth, or to treat people suffering from nausea due to chemotherapy.

Acupuncture's effectiveness in chronic diseases such as asthma and hay fever – over the placebo effects (see box on page 200) – needs further investigation. Some studies seem to suggest that acupuncture alleviates asthma. A review of several studies suggested that acupuncture may produce some benefit in an acute asthma attack, but that the benefit is less marked than that produced by a bronchodilator.[7] Nevertheless, some researchers regard many of these studies of being 'rather poor quality'. They suggest that, overall, there is not sufficient evidence to make any recommendations about acupuncture's role in asthma treatment.[1]

The British Acupuncture Council (BAaC),★ British Medical Acupuncture Society★ and Acupuncture Association of Chartered Physiotherapists★ ensure that practitioners are trained and accredited. Many GPs now offer acupuncture – usually only for pain relief. All registered practitioners will use sterile needles. However, there is no statutory need to be registered and anyone can call themselves an acupuncturist.

Alexander technique

At around the end of the nineteenth century, the Australian actor Frederick Matthias Alexander began experiencing serious voice problems, which doctors could not alleviate. Alexander noticed that when he spoke he pulled his head back. He also inhaled when he began to speak – this compressed his vocal cords. By changing the way he held his head and neck he found he could improve his breathing. This observation led to the Alexander technique.

Alexander argued that if you habitually adopt postures for which the body is not designed, your muscles and nerves are not going to work correctly. If your nerves do not work properly, he suggested, neither do the organs they serve. So Alexander teachers re-educate people about correct postures. This restores the body's normal functions. As a result, some teachers of the Alexander technique say that people with asthma who practise the technique find breathing easier. It certainly seems logical that better posture could help you breathe better. Indeed, some studies of healthy volunteers suggest that the Alexander technique can improve respiratory function.

On the other hand, review of the evidence for the Alexander technique failed to find any well-designed controlled trials that showed that it improved chronic asthma in people who were well controlled by their medication, either compared to another intervention or to no treatment.[8] But, as mentioned earlier, a lack of evidence doesn't necessarily mean that the therapy is ineffective; it's possible that the appropriate studies haven't been performed. So there is a need for well-designed studies to see whether the Alexander technique improves the symptoms of chronic asthma and reduces people's need for medication.

Nevertheless, the Alexander technique is unlikely to do you any harm and may aid relaxation. But you need to be committed to the practice. You cannot teach yourself the Alexander technique, and teachers can take 30 or more sessions to re-educate your body. Moreover, you will need to practise the technique every day. The Society of Teachers of the Alexander Technique (STAT)* is the main umbrella organisation in the UK. STAT has around 1,130 teachers who have completed a three-year training course and are insured.

Buteyko method

The Buteyko method aims to recondition and normalise breathing using special exercises and lifestyle changes. And an increasing number of studies suggest that some people with asthma may benefit from Buteyko.

For example, one study[9] from Nottingham of people with asthma found that performing the Buteyko breathing technique for six months improved symptoms and reduced bronchodilator use by an average of two puffs a day. However, FEV_1 (see Chapter 6), exacerbations or inhaled steroid use did not change.

An Australian study[10] assessing Buteyko drew broadly similar results. Neither daily peak flow nor FEV_1 changed. However, those practising Buteyko reduced their use of both $beta_2$-agonists and the dose of inhaled steroids – the latter by 49 per cent. They were also less likely to hyperventilate.

So there is some evidence that Buteyko may improve asthma symptoms. Indeed, some people may be able to reduce their use of asthma medication. It is important, however, to discuss any change in your drugs regimen with your doctor first.

Herbalism

The Chinese and Indians recognised lung diseases similar to asthma as long ago as 1,550 BC. The Chinese used the herb *Ma Huang* (also called ephedra), which contains the beta$_2$-agonist ephedrine. (However, ephedra also seems to cause potentially serious side-effects – see below.) During the early nineteenth century, asthmatics smoked thorn-apple leaves. The active ingredient, stramonium, was also the main ingredient in the popular Potter's Asthma Cure. Stramonium is a member of a group of drugs called anticholinergics, which dilate bronchi through a different mechanism from the beta$_2$-agonists. Around the same time, people with asthma took belladonna's active ingredient – atropine, another anticholinergic – and drank strong coffee. We now know that coffee contains natural xanthines similar to theophylline (see Chapter 7 for more about the drugs used in conventional asthma treatment).

Worldwide, about four billion people rely on plants as their main source of medicines. Herbalism is also popular in the UK, and while no one seriously disputes that some herbs are effective, some doctors question their safety. They point out that some herbs contain potent, even toxic, chemicals. Heroin, cocaine and cannabis are derived from plants, for example. At high doses some plants – those containing stramonium and atropine, for instance – are poisons. And there are concerns that ephedra could be associated with severe side-effects, including heart attacks, strokes, seizures and even death.[11] Moreover, some studies link Chinese herbs with damage to the kidneys, liver and heart, as well as hypersensitivity reactions (see Chapter 12). In at least one case, a herbal treatment for eczema has been linked to a death.[12]

Herbalism's critics also argue that few herbal remedies undergo the same systematic and scientifically rigorous long-term safety testing as pharmaceutical drugs. On the other hand, herbal remedies have had hundreds or thousands of years of use, which may offer some assurance of the herbs' safety. Nevertheless, serious side-effects can still occur with herbal preparations used for millennia – as the concerns about ephedra illustrate.

Another reason for caution is that there is no control over a preparation's composition. Indeed, a *Which?* report in 2001[13] revealed that some Chinese herbal preparations contained potent levels of steroids. So it is important to seek treatment from a reputable, well-qualified herbalist (see the end of this section for contact organisations).

Despite these concerns, CAM practitioners advocate several herbal treatments from various traditions – including Chinese, Indian and Western – to alleviate asthma and other allergic diseases. But there is relatively little scientific evidence that herbal treatments benefit asthma.[1] Again, this may reflect the fact that these traditional treatments have not been assessed in formal clinical studies. Nevertheless, only one of three well-designed studies suggested that a herbal remedy improved lung function in people with asthma.

On the other hand, there is some evidence that herbal treatments work for eczema: in scientific trials, Chinese medicine has had some successes. Not all studies confirm the benefits in atopic dermatitis described below,[14] although ethnic differences may account for this.[12] Chinese herbalists believe that asthma and other illnesses arise from disruption in the flow of chi (see pages 205–7). This differs in everyone, so Chinese herbalists tailor the mix of herbs to the patient. Treatment aims to rebalance chi to restore the balance of energy in the body. You will probably be given a mixture of herbs and asked to prepare a drink several times a day.

In one study, 47 children with extensive atopic dermatitis received a Chinese herbal mixture for eight weeks. Erythema (skin redness) decreased by 51 per cent in those that received the herbal mixture compared with a 6 per cent fall in the placebo group. Damage to the skin surface declined by 63 per cent in the group taking herbs and 6 per cent in the placebo users. In another study, 40 adults with difficult-to-manage atopic dermatitis received the herbal mixture. Erythema and damage to the skin surface improved by 46 and 49 per cent *more* respectively in those taking the herbs compared with placebo.[15] Other research found that a similar herbal mixture seemed to blunt some aspects of the immunological changes that underlie atopic dermatitis: for example, levels of IgE declined (see Chapter 1). The immunological changes parallelled the improvement in erythema and damage to the surface of the skin[16].

Remember that some herbs may interact with conventional medicines prescribed by your doctor. So you must tell your doctor and pharmacist if you are using herbal remedies, and your herbalist needs to know which conventional drugs you are taking. Similarly, you should let the doctor know if you are taking a herbal medicine before you have a skin prick or other diagnostic test. Some herbs can contain anti-inflammatory chemicals that could influence the results.

If you are, or plan to be, pregnant, or want to use herbs to treat a child, always consult a qualified medical herbalist first. However, as with most drugs, you should avoid taking herbs during pregnancy. The National Institute of Medical Herbalists (NIMH)★ Register of Chinese Herbal Medicine can help you find a local practitioner.

Homeopathy

Homeopathy is one of the most popular CAMs in the UK. Indeed, it accounts for around half of all CAM treatments on the NHS. But whether it works is controversial. *Health Which?* reported in June 2002[17] that researchers from the University of York concluded that 'there's currently insufficient evidence from randomised controlled trials to recommend [homeopathy] for any specific condition'. But, again, the lack of evidence may reflect the fact that most studies are poorly designed rather than a lack of effectiveness per se.

On the one hand, many people find that homeopathy alleviates allergic symptoms – and there are some scientific studies to support this (see below), especially in allergic rhinitis. On the other hand, most scientists are sceptical about homeopathy's claims, especially as it challenges some of the foundations of Western medicine.

The word homeopathy derives from the Greek *homoios*, meaning 'like', and *pathos*, meaning 'suffering'. This reflects homeopathy's aim to work with the body through treating 'like with like'. Homeopathy's advocates point out that this principal isn't as unusual as it may sound. For example, the bark of the cinchona tree alleviates symptoms in patients with malaria, but when healthy people take cinchona bark, they develop side-effects that are similar to malaria. And conventional vaccines are based on the idea that a small amount of a micro-organism confers protection against subsequent infection. But there's a fundamental difference between these examples and homeopathy: there are widely accepted mechanisms through which cinchona and vaccines work.

To understand why homeopathy is so controversial, we need to take a brief detour into the history of the therapy. In 1811, the German physician Dr Samuel Hahnemann was disillusioned. He had trained in orthodox medicine, but his treatments often did more harm than good. Hahnemann believed that the symptoms of disease reflected the body's efforts to overcome illness – in direct opposition to conventional doctors, who believed that illnesses caused the symptoms. Hahnemann abandoned his practice to experiment with other ways of healing.

Hahnemann experimented with single substances from plants, animals and minerals. To avoid side-effects, he diluted the substances in water and alcohol, which he mixed by vigorous shaking. Remarkably, Hahnemann found that the more dilute a substance became, the more potent its therapeutic action. On the other hand, substances that produced dissimilar side-effects in healthy people to those being treated in people with the disease had no effect on those symptoms. Hahnemann called his method of diluting chemicals 'potentisation' and the serial dilutions 'potencies'. The high degree of dilution allows homeopaths to use poisons such as arsenic, morphine and cocaine to treat patients, without causing side-effects. Homeopaths believe that potentisation can also transform sand, salt and charcoal into potent remedies – as long as they are tailored for the right person suffering from the right disease.

Potentisation contributes to some doctors' accusations that homeopathy is biologically implausible. The formulations used are so dilute that the patient is unlikely to receive a single molecule of the 'active' ingredient. Moreover, the claim that a treatment becomes more potent as dilution increases goes against a fundamental principle of medical science. Biologically active substances tend to follow a 'dose–response' relationship: below a certain dose, a drug produces no effect. Above this threshold, response increases until it reaches a plateau, after which increasing the dose has no further effect. Homeopathy turns the dose–response relationship on its head.

The style of some 'classical' homeopathic consultations further undermines many conventional doctors' belief in homeopathy. Instead of enquiring only about symptoms, lifestyle and medical and family history, classical homeopathic healers also seek to determine whether you are musical, scientific or artistic; sulky or rapidly angered, and so on. Classical homeopaths even note their clients' hair and eye colour and pay attention to their hopes and fears. In this way, the therapist develops a detailed picture of the patient and matches a remedy to this profile. Cynics suggest that this intense interest shown to patients could increase the power of suggestion and enhance the placebo effect (see page 200).

Despite this scepticism, there is evidence that homeopathy may work in some people with certain allergic diseases. For example, a study published in 1986[18] compared the effects of a homeopathic preparation of grass seed pollen and a placebo in 144 hay fever sufferers. Neither the doctors nor the patients knew which the latter received. Nevertheless, patients who received the homeopathic preparation reported fewer symptoms – and the doctors agreed that the patients benefited from homeopathy.

In a more recent study,[19] researchers treated 51 people suffering from perennial allergic rhinitis, using either a homoeopathic preparation of the main inhaled allergen or placebo. Those that received homeopathy showed improved nasal airflow that was similar to that produced by nasal steroids. The people taking homeopathy also reported a greater improvement in symptoms than the placebo group. Finally, 30 per cent of the homeopathy group and 7 per cent of those receiving placebo reported that their symptoms initially worsened. This phenomenon – called 'proving' or the 'healing reaction' – is characteristic of homeopathic remedies.

Taking the above and other studies together, symptoms of allergic rhinitis improved by an average of 28 per cent among homeopathy users compared to 3 per cent in the placebo group. So there is some evidence that homeopathy may alleviate allergic rhinitis.

Overall, however, there is not enough evidence to reliably assess whether homeopathy is effective in asthma. In 1994, the research group that performed the 1986 study reported that homeopathy alleviated asthma more effectively than placebo.[20] Subjects who took the homeopathic preparation reported fewer and less intense symptoms – the benefits persisted for eight weeks and lung function also improved. Nevertheless, this result was relatively modest compared to the effect of modern anti-asthma medications.

Other results are mixed. Several studies that did not use a placebo control suggested that homeopathy benefits asthma. Better-controlled studies, however, are less convincing. In classical home-opathy, treatment is individualised to the patients' characteristics (see above). One study[21] assessed the effect of classical homeopathy, compared to placebo, over a year, in children with mild to moderate asthma aged between 5 and 15 years. The children were already taking inhaled beta$_2$-agonists and steroids (see Chapter 7). Adding homeopathic treatment did not improve peak flow or reduce medication use, symptoms, days off school or other measures of asthma.

A further study[22] enrolled 242 people with asthma who also showed positive skin-prick results for house dust mites (see Chapters 2 and 3). The subjects received oral homeopathy or placebo and were assessed over 16 weeks. In general, no differences emerged between placebo and homeopathy. On the other hand, those treated with homeopathy showed alternating deterioration and improvement. The researchers admitted that the difference in the pattern of response between the two groups is 'unexplained'. This may hint, however, that homeopathy produces a biological effect.

Your GP may be able to refer you to a homeopathic hospital or a local qualified homeopath for treatment on the NHS. About 1,000 NHS doctors practise homeopathy.[23] About half of these are registered with the Faculty of Homeopathy,* established by an Act of Parliament to train and register practitioners. The Society of Homeopaths* has some 1,500 members registered, who have undergone a three-year course and are fully insured. You can also buy homeopathic remedies from chemists and health food shops. However, these off-the-shelf remedies are not specifically tailored to each person and are unlikely to be as effective as bespoke therapy.

Hypnotherapy

For centuries, hypnotism was dismissed a stage trick, with its benefits confined to the gullible. In the late eighteenth century Franz Mesmer, a Viennese doctor, put large numbers of people into trances, calling the technique 'mesmerism'. His theatrical presentation alienated the medical community, however. Then, towards the end of the nineteenth century, the French physician Liébeault offered to treat people for free – provided they allowed him to hypnotise them. After putting his peasant volunteers into a hypnotic trance, Liébeault used hypnotism to suggest that their headaches, stomach aches and other pains would resolve. His success rate was high enough for his fame to spread. Liébeault is considered the founder of modern hypnotherapy.

The technique was brought to the UK in the late nineteenth century by the Manchester surgeon James Braid, who coined the term hypnotism (from the Greek *hypnos*, meaning 'sleep'). Before the introduction of chloroform, major operations – including amputations and the removal of large tumours – were sometimes performed under hypnosis, apparently without patients experiencing pain. Although widely accepted among their Continental colleagues, members of the British medical profession refused to take hypnotism seriously.

The tide changed in the 1950s, when the *British Medical Journal* reported that hypnotism cured ichthyosis – a disfiguring disease where the skin appears rough and horny. A young boy was put into a hypnotic trance and told which areas of his skin would clear. These areas became almost normal. In 1955, hypnosis began to be accepted as a valid medical treatment for certain conditions. Most doctors now accept that hypnosis alleviates stress and may help some types of chronic pain and some addictions, including smoking.

Against this background, researchers reviewed the growing body of evidence suggesting that hypnosis improves symptoms in some people with asthma.[24] People who are susceptible to hypnosis, are treated by an experienced hypnotherapist, participate in several sessions, and reinforce the sessions with autohypnosis (self-hypnosis) seemed to benefit most. The researchers added that children seemed to respond especially well. Nevertheless, they suggested that further, larger well-designed studies are needed to fully characterise the benefits of hypnosis in asthma. There is also some evidence that hypnotherapy can benefit atopic dermatitis and urticaria,[25] although again more research is needed.

Not everyone is easily hypnotised. Even stage hypnotists pick their subjects carefully. For it to work, you have to want to be hypnotised. The best subjects tend to be people who immerse themselves in the imaginary worlds of books, films and plays and strongly identify with imaginary characters. Those who are motivated and keen to change their lives are more likely to be easily hypnotised than people who like to be strongly in control or have conditions such as anorexia and obsessive-compulsive disorder.

No one really understands how hypnotism works. It is clear that, despite its name, hypnotism is not a form of sleep. Most people feel tired, lethargic and drowsy during hypnosis. However, although the brain's electrical activity changes during hypnosis, the alterations do not resemble sleep. Indeed, electrical activity in the brain suggests the subject is fully awake during hypnosis. According to one favoured theory, the brain shuts off nerves supplying sensory information. The subject's attention becomes highly selective and he or she tends to show reduced mental planning – instead waiting for instructions. Certainly, during hypnosis subjects become very relaxed and less critical – which is why stage hypnotists can make people act as dogs or chickens. But it's also why hypnosis can help reduce stress and may alleviate asthma. In all cases the subject seems willing to give up conscious control voluntarily and becomes highly suggestible.

For lists of qualified hypnotists contact the Central Register of Advanced Hypnotherapists (CRAH)* or the National Register of Hypnotherapists and Psychotherapists.*

Meditation

Like yoga (see page 218) and the Buteyko method (see page 208), meditation often emphasises correct breathing. Transcendental Meditation (TM), developed in the 1960s by the Maharishi Mahesh Yogi, is the most-studied form, and there is some evidence from clinical studies that it directly improves asthma as well as offering a number of non-specific health benefits, such as countering stress.

Back in 1975, researchers performed a six-month study[26] that compared two groups: one of which followed TM and one that did not meditate. After three months, the TM group stopped and those that had not been meditating began. After three weeks, the meditators' asthma symptoms worsened – possibly because meditation made them more aware of their breathing. After this the symptoms began to improve. After six months the meditators reported fewer symptoms than before starting the experiment and showed improved lung function. Three of the five people who were on oral steroids at the start of the study were able to stop taking them; though others tended to use the same amount of asthma medication. In other words, TM is an addition to, rather than a replacement for, anti-asthma drugs. Further studies are needed to confirm these results and quantify the benefits.

A more recent study[27] assessed a form of meditation based on yogic principles. The study enrolled people who had asthma symptoms despite taking moderate to high doses of inhaled steroids. Those who meditated showed less airway hyper-responsiveness than those who did not. Mood also improved to a greater extent in the yoga group. Two months after treatment ended, however, there was no difference between those in the meditation group and those in the control group. So, while further studies are needed to fully determine the benefits, there seems to be some evidence that meditation benefits people with asthma.

Learning meditation

People of all ages, backgrounds and religions meditate. Classically, meditation involves sitting serenely on a mat with your eyes closed and your legs crossed, focusing on your breathing or a special saying (called a 'mantra') for 20 to 30 minutes a couple of times a day. TM uses slightly shorter sessions of 15 to 20 minutes, two or three times a day. While this may seem a considerable time commitment in a busy life, meditators argue that taking 40 to 60 minutes a day to meditate helps you achieve more with less effort. After a while, meditation becomes part of your routine, and can also be a 'coping strategy' that you can call on when stressed.

To learn meditation correctly, it's advisable to receive instruction from a teacher (see overleaf), although you could get a feel for meditation by trying it for yourself, as follows, before investing time and (in some cases) money on a course.

- Find somewhere quiet. Beginners find meditation especially difficult where there are too many distractions.
- Sit comfortably. This doesn't need to be the full cross-legged 'lotus' position – a chair is fine. You'll need to sit still for about 20 minutes without the distractions of cramps and other aches.

- Now breathe deeply. Meditation teachers emphasise that most people tend to breathe into their chests instead of their abdomens. By concentrating, you can learn to breathe slowly and evenly in highly stressful situations – maybe even during an acute asthma attack.
- Now focus your attention. TM uses a mantra – a personal phrase or saying given to you by your teacher. But you could use a common mantra such as 'Om', or choose your own (it does not have to be exotic – any simple non-emotive word will do, even if it's nonsense). Other techniques encourage 'mindful meditation', where you maintain moment-to-moment awareness of the motion of your breath in and out of your nose and mouth. You can also focus on a candle flame, crystal or icon. These all have the same effect: they concentrate your mind and exclude distractions.
- Maintaining concentration for 20 minutes is far harder than it sounds. You will probably find that your mind wanders off. Just accept these ramblings and re-focus your attention on the subject. Try not to be annoyed with yourself.

Finding a meditation teacher

Transcendental Meditation★ is taught across the UK. If you decide TM is for you, you will probably go to four sessions on consecutive days and a further session three months later. TM is not the only type of meditation – so there is some choice of courses and you should be able to find one that suits you and your pocket. Some can be expensive, while others ask only for a donation of what you feel you can afford or may be free. The Buddhist Society UK★ can put you in touch with teachers of traditional Buddhist or Zen meditation. Finally, meditation is an integral part of yoga. Contact the British Wheel of Yoga★ for further information.

Yoga

Yoga was first practised 5,000 years ago in India. The practice reached Britain during the Victorian era, but did not really catch on until the 1960s. The several types of yoga practised today bring millions of people around the world inner peace, helps keep them fit, relieves stress and improves health. Yoga is far removed from the image of forcing your body into strange positions in a draughty church hall. Traditional Indian yoga is a complete system that helps you manage your life, although many teachers in the UK tend to focus on only one particular aspect of the system. Even if yoga doesn't directly benefit allergic diseases, it can certainly make you feel a lot better. And there is some evidence that the general improvement arising from yoga can help alleviate asthma symptoms.

In common with some other CAMs, yoga conceives of all aspects of your life – consciousness, mind, energy and body – as intertwined. Yoga aims to harmonise these aspects: the Sanskrit root of the word yoga means 'to unite'. Yoga seeks to achieve this unity in three ways.

Posture

Yoga is perhaps best known for the postures that impose some control over our unruly bodies. There are some 80 of these postures. Known as 'asanas', they are more than physical exercises. Correctly performed, asanas involve mental control, correct breathing and using your body with minimum effort and tension. The postures gently stretch and contract muscles and joints. This allows you to move more freely and improves stamina, flexibility and strength. Teachers claim that asanas train the mind and raise consciousness.

Mental balance

Yoga teachers assert that regular practice can raise consciousness. This means, for example, that yoga may bolster your stress defences and may help reduce your fears – perhaps about future asthma or anaphylactic attacks. We worry about many events that have not happened yet instead of devoting our energy to the present. Yoga and meditation help us live in the present.

Breath control

Yoga emphasises correct breathing. When you are tense, your breaths tend to be shallow and centre on the upper chest. By performing breathing exercises – pranayama – that retrain and learn to control the breath. Yoga teachers believe that breath control allows them to regulate their physical and mental processes and helps them attain the ultimate goal of yoga – self-enlightenment.

More prosaically, by practising yoga you should become more aware of your lungs and how they feel. This may mean that you are more likely to be able to detect a change in your asthma symptoms. As we've seen (see Chapter 6), people with asthma do not always accurately perceive their lung function. Yoga is not a substitute for your peak flow meter, however.

There is some evidence that yoga can improve asthma. For example, researchers have found that people with asthma who practised yoga experienced fewer attacks, used fewer drugs and showed improved peak flow compared to controls.[28] Several other studies using yoga and other breathing exercises show similar results. One of these found that yoga benefited patients when used in addition to drugs for asthma.[29]

While these results are promising, you should not change your asthma regimen without talking to your doctor first. Provided you only reduce your medication under medical supervision, it's quite possible that yoga and other breathing exercises could help your asthma. But further studies are needed to fully determine the benefits associated with yoga.

Finding a yoga class

You should perform yoga in a quiet, warm, well-ventilated room. Wear comfortable, light clothes and do not practise on a full stomach. You will need to attend classes to learn yoga correctly and the teacher should be well trained. A report in *Health Which?* in August 2003[30] highlighted a shortage of trained yoga teachers. The report suggested asking for details of the teacher's qualification – and checking that his or her qualifications are up to date – as well as asking to see the instructors' insurance certificate. It also warned that large classes 'can be a recipe for disaster' and suggested sitting at the back of a class before joining. A poor instructor may leave the class struggling to follow instructions and may not individually correct pupils. Teachers of Iyengar yoga must have practised this form of yoga for at least five years, with three years of training, before they can teach.[23]

Apart from attending classes you must be prepared to set aside some time to practise each day – ideally 20 to 30 minutes. Be prepared not to see instant benefits. It takes time to learn how to train your body. A wide range of books and videos offers a basic understanding of yoga and its benefits. The British Wheel of Yoga★ can provide further details. The Yoga for Health Foundation★ runs yoga retreats. Your library or adult education centre may also have details of local courses.

Chapter summary

Complementary and alternative medicine is increasingly popular among people who have allergic diseases. There seems to be no validated use for any of the alternative diagnostic tests for allergies. Few of the treatments advocated for asthma and other allergic diseases have been well studied in scientifically rigorous studies. But there are indications that some might benefit some people with certain allergic diseases, although further studies are needed. Nevertheless, used alongside conventional management, CAM can help many people suffering from allergic diseases.

As researchers have noted, using CAM can help people with allergies feel more empowered, more actively involved in decision making and more in control of their disease.[1] And that is the whole ethos of this book.

Glossary

Acaricides Chemicals that kill house dust mites

Acute Rapid onset of symptoms or a condition

Allergen A substance that triggers an allergic reaction

Allergy Symptoms that arise when an oversensitive immune system reacts strongly to a substance that most people find benign. Allergies can develop in, for example, the skin (eczema), lungs (asthma) or nose and eyes (allergic rhinitis and conjunctivitis respectively)

Anaphylaxis A severe, potentially life-threatening, allergic reaction

Anaphylactoid A reaction that resembles anaphylaxis but that is not allergic

Angioedema Swelling of tissues beneath the skin

Antibodies Proteins – such as IgE – circulating in the blood that stimulate the immune system

Antihistamine A drug that antagonises – blocks – histamine

Anti-inflammatories Also called 'preventers'. Drugs that reduce inflammation. Steroids are one widely used class of anti-inflammatory drug

Atopic/atopy Of people: a genetic tendency to develop IgE-mediated allergic conditions. Of a disease: IgE-mediated

B-lymphocytes White blood cells, formed in the bone marrow, that produce antibodies and protect the body from invasion by foreign proteins

Beta$_2$-agonists Drugs that bind to beta$_2$-receptors on the muscle cells surrounding the bronchi, leading to relaxation. Beta$_2$-agonists are bronchodilators

Bronchi The airways in the lung that become inflamed in asthma. The trachea divides into two major bronchi and then sub-divides, eventually leading to bronchioles

Bronchioles The 20,000 to 80,000 small airways in the lung that become inflamed in asthma

Bronchoconstriction Contraction of the muscle surrounding the bronchi, leading to narrowing of the airways. May also be called bronchospasm

Bronchodilators Also called 'relievers'. Drugs, such as the beta$_2$-agonists, that open the bronchi

Bronchospasm See bronchoconstriction

Chronic Long-lasting symptoms or condition

Compliance The extent to which the patient follows the doctor's instructions (usually refers to drugs); also called accordance

Conjunctivitis Inflammation of the conjunctiva – the layer of cells that covers the whites of the eyes and the insides of the eyelids

Corticosteroids (Steroids). A type of hormone that dampens inflammation. The body produces some corticosteroids naturally

Cromolyns Drugs that 'stabilise' mast cells, preventing them from degranulating. An example is sodium cromoglycate (also spelled 'cromoglicate')

Cross-react Many people allergic to one allergen also react to another. So, for example, people with food allergies often cross-react to several different foods

Dermatitis Eczema

Dander Small pieces of hair and skin shed by animals

Enzymes Specialised proteins that speed up chemical reactions

Exacerbation A worsening of symptoms

Erythema Skin redness

FEV$_1$ Forced expiratory volume in one second – a measure of lung function

FVC Forced vital capacity. The total volume of air expelled after a full breath in – a measure of lung function

Hapten The combination of a drug (or its metabolite) and the protein to which it has bonded. Haptens can act as allergens

Histamine An inflammatory mediator released from mast cells

Hives See urticaria

Hyper-responsiveness When the bronchi of people with asthma are excessively sensitive or 'twitchy'. These people are more likely to develop bronchoconstriction

Hypotension Fall in blood pressure

Hypertension Increase in blood pressure; when chronic this increases the risk of, for example, heart disease and stroke

IgE Immunoglobulin E. The antibody responsible for atopic symptoms. Many allergies are mediated (caused) by IgE

Immune response The reaction of the body's defences (the immune system) to an invading organism or infection

Immunotherapy A treatment in which people with allergies are injected with increasing amounts of the allergen, which can 'switch off' the immune response to that allergen

Inflammation A local protective response following injury

Inflammatory mediators Mediators that co-ordinate the immune response

Larynx voicebox

Leukotrienes A type of inflammatory mediator. One particular leukotriene plays a major role in driving bronchoconstriction in asthma

Lacrimation Tear production

Mast cells A type of white blood cell. Masts cell contain granules that contain inflammatory mediators, including histamine. Antibodies bind to the mast cells and trigger them to degranulate, releasing a 'cocktail' of inflammatory mediators. The binding also leads to the production of other mediators

Mediators Chemicals in the body that stimulate or inhibit other cells

Metabolites The chemicals produced when the body uses, for example, enzymes to break down drugs

NSAIDs (non-steroidal anti-inflammatory drugs) A group of drugs, which includes aspirin and ibuprofen, widely used to treat mild pain and inflammatory diseases such as arthritis. In some people with asthma, NSAIDs or related natural chemicals, called salicylates, may provoke an attack

Oedema Swelling

Peak expiratory flow rate See peak flow

Peak flow The maximum flow rate of air breathed out – the most widely used measure of lung function

Perennial Year-round

Placebo A substance that appears the same as a drug but which lacks the active ingredient

Preventers See anti-inflammatories

Prostate The gland that produces some of the ejaculate in men. It lies at the base of the bladder, surrounding the urethra (the tube urine passes through)

Pruritis – itching

Relievers See bronchodilators

Remodelling In asthma, structural changes to the lungs caused by prolonged inflammation. For example, the airway walls thicken, and the bronchi become scarred and can be blocked with mucus

Rhinitis Nasal inflammation

Rhinoconjunctivitis Combination of nasal symptoms and conjunctivitis

Rhinnorhoea Dripping nose

Salicylates A group of chemicals that includes NSAIDs

Seasonal allergic rhinitis hay fever

Sensitised When the immune system is primed to respond to an allergen. The person is likely to develop allergic symptoms next time he or she is exposed to that allergen

Steroids See corticosteroids

Systemic A widespread reaction – one that occurs in several sites throughout the body

T-lymphocytes (T-cells.) White blood cells that co-ordinate the immune response. There are several broad classes of T-cell. Cytotoxic T-cells destroy invading bacteria and viruses. T-helper cells stimulate B-lymphocytes to produce antibodies to pathogens and allergens. Memory T-cells help the body respond to specific pathogens and allergens it has encountered before

Topical Applied to the outside of the body – for example, to the eye or skin

Trachea windpipe

Upper respiratory tract The nose, mouth, trachea and larynx

Urticaria Also known as 'hives'. Red, itchy bumps on the skin

Bibliography

You can find many of the following papers on the Internet, using the common search engines or PubMed (www.nebi.nlm.nih.gov/PubMed), an electronic medical library. Many libraries now offer Internet access and the staff should be able to help you track the paper down.

Chapter 1

End notes

1 Karlen, A. 1996. *Plague's Progress*. Indigo
2 Hollinger, M.A. 2003. *Introduction to Pharmacology*. Taylor & Francis
3 Royal College of Physicians. June 2003. *Allergy: The Unmet Need – A blueprint for better patient care*
4 Ewan, P.W. 1998. Anaphylaxis. *BMJ*, 316, 1,442–5
5 Linna, O., Kokkonen, J., Lahtela, P. et al. 1992. Ten-year prognosis for generalized infantile eczema. *Acta Paediatr*, 81, 1,013–6
6 Arshad, S.H., Kurukulaaratchy, R.J., Fenn, M. et al. 2002. Rhinitis in 10-year-old children and early life risk factors for its development. *Acta Paediatr*, 91, 1,334–8
7 Strachan, D.P., Wong, H.J. and Spector, T.D. 2001. Concordance and interrelationship of atopic diseases and markers of allergic sensitization among adult female twins. *J Allergy Clin Immunol*, 108, 901–7
8 Skadhauge, L.R., Christensen, K., Kyvik, K.O. et al. 1999. Genetic and environmental influence on asthma: a population-based study of 11,688 Danish twin pairs. *Eur Respir J*, 13, 8–14
9 Austin, J.B., Kaur, B., Anderson, H.R., Burr. M. 1999. Hay fever, eczema, and wheeze: a nationwide UK study (ISAAC, international study of asthma and allergies in childhood). *Arch Dis Child*, 81, 225–30
10 Beasley, R., Lai, C.K., Crane, J. et al. 1998. The video questionnaire: one approach to the identification of the asthmatic phenotype. *Clin Exp Allergy*, Suppl 11, 8–12, 32–6
11 Aberg, N., Hesselmar, B., Aberg, B. et al. 1995. Increase of asthma, allergic rhinitis and eczema in Swedish school children between 1979 and 1991. *Clin Exp Allergy*, 25, 815–9

12   Miescher, S.M. and Vogel, M. 2002. Molecular aspects of allergy. *Molecular Aspects of Medicine*, 23, 413–62

13   Yazdanbakhsh, M., van den Biggelaara, M. and Maizelsb, R.M. 2001. Th$_2$ responses without atopy: immunoregulation in chronic helminth infections and reduced allergic disease. *Trends in Immunology*, 22, 372–7

14   Hilliquin, P., Allanore, Y., Coste, J. et al. 2000. Reduced incidence and prevalence of atopy in rheumatoid arthritis. Results of a case-control study. *Rheumatology*, 39, 1,020–6

General

Bowry, T. R. 1984. *Immunology Simplified*. Oxford University Press

Klein, J. and Horejsi, V. 1997. *Immunology*. Blackwell

Lösel, R., Feuring, M. and Wehling, M. 2003. Non-genomic aldosterone action: from the cell membrane to human physiology. *Journal of Steroid Biochemistry & Molecular Biology*, 83, 167–71

Chapter 2

End notes

1   Vieths, S., Scheurer, S. and Ballmer-Weber, B. 2002. Current understanding of cross-reactivity of food allergens and pollen. *Ann N Y Acad Sci*, 964, 47–68

2   Royal College of Physicians. June 2003. *Allergy: The Unmet Need – A blueprint for better patient care*

3   Emberlin, J., Mullins, J., Corden, J., Millington, W. et al. 1997. The trend to earlier birch pollen seasons in the UK: a biotic response to changes in weather conditions. *Grana*, 36, 29–33

4   Lomborg, B. 2001. *The Skeptical Environmentalist*. Cambridge University Press

5   *Air Purifiers*. Which?, March 2003, pp 28–9

6   Codina, R., Lockey, R.F., Diwadkar, R. et al. 2003. Disodium octaborate tetrahydrate (DOT) application and vacuum cleaning, a combined strategy to control house dust mites. *Allergy*, 58, 318–24

7   Mihrshahi, S., Marks, G.B., Criss, S. et al. 2003. Effectiveness of an intervention to reduce house dust mite allergen levels in children's beds. *Allergy*, 58, 784–9

8   Linneberg, A., Nielsen, N.H., Madsen, F. et al. 2003. Pets in the home and the development of pet allergy in adulthood. The Copenhagen Allergy Study. *Allergy*, 58, 21–6

9   Heissenhuber, A., Heinrich, J., Fahlbusch, B. et al. 2003. Health impacts of second-hand exposure to cat allergen Fel d 1 in infants. *Allergy*, 58, 154–7

10 Golden, D.B. 2003. Stinging insect allergy. *Am Fam Physician*, 5, 67, 2,541–6

11 Ahmed, D.D., Sobczak, S.C. and Yunginger, J.W. 2003. Occupational allergies caused by latex. *Immunol Allergy Clin North Am*, 23, 205–19

12 Edlich, R.F., Woodard, C.R., Hill, L.G. et al. 2003. Latex allergy: a life-threatening epidemic for scientists, healthcare personnel, and their patients. *J Long Term Eff Med Implants*, 13, 11–9

13 Nettis, E., Dambra, P., Soccio, A.L., et al. 2003. Latex hypersensitivity: relationship with positive prick test and patch test responses among hairdressers. *Allergy*, 58, 57–61

14 Silverman, R.A., Boudreaux, E.D., Woodruff, P.G. et al. 2003. Cigarette smoking among asthmatic adults presenting to 64 emergency departments. *Chest*, 123, 1,472–9

15 Harty, S.B., Sheridan, A., Howell, F. et al. 2003. Wheeze, eczema and rhinitis in 6–7 year old Irish schoolchildren. *Ir Med J*, 96, 102–4

16 Larsson, M.L., Loit, H.M., Meren, M. et al. 2003. Passive smoking and respiratory symptoms in the FinEsS study. *Eur Respir J*, 21, 672–6

17 Jang, A-S., Yeum, C-H. and Son, M-H. 2003. Epidemiologic evidence of a relationship between airway hyperresponsiveness and exposure to polluted air. *Allergy*, 58, 585–8

General

Asthma. Health Which?, April 2002, pp 30–1

Fighting Hayfever. Health Which?, April 1997, pp 52–3

Help with Hayfever. Which?, May 2001, pp 46–9

Valenta, R., Duchene, M., Ebner, C. et al. 1992. Profilins constitute a novel family of functional plant pan-allergens. *J Exp Med*, 175, 377–85

Chapter 3

1 Rusznak, C. and Davies, R.J. 1998. Diagnosing allergy. *BMJ*, 316, 686–9

2 Fiocchi, A., Bouygue, G.R., Restani, P. et al. 2002. Accuracy of skin prick tests in IgE-mediated adverse reactions to bovine proteins. *Ann Allergy Asthma Immunol*, 89 (6 Suppl 1), 26–32

3 Pirker, C., Misic, A., Brinkmeier, T. et al. 2002. Tetrazepam drug sensitivity – usefulness of the patch test. *Contact Dermatitis*, 47, 135–8

4 Modjtahedi, S.P. and Maibach, H.I. 2002. Ethnicity as a possible endogenous factor in irritant contact dermatitis: comparing the irritant response among Caucasians, blacks and Asians. *Contact Dermatitis*, 47, 272–8

5 Scadding, G.K. 2001. Non-allergic rhinitis: diagnosis and management. *Curr Opin Allergy Clin Immunol*, 1, 15–20

6 Baker, J.C., Duncanson, R.C., Tunnicliffe, W.S. et al. 2000. Development of a standardized methodology for double-blind, placebo-controlled food challenge in patients with brittle asthma and perceived food intolerance. *J Am Diet Assoc*, 100, 1,361–7

7 Kotaniemi-Syrjanen, A., Reijonen, T.M., Romppanen, J. et al. 2003. Allergen-specific immunoglobulin E antibodies in wheezing infants: the risk for asthma in later childhood. *Pediatrics*, 111, E255–61

Chapter 4

1   Ewan, P.W. 1998. Anaphylaxis. *BMJ*, 316, 1,442–5
2   Sheikh, A. and Alves, B. 2000. Hospital admissions for acute anaphylaxis: time trend study. *BMJ*, 320, 1,441
3   Shadick, N.A., Liang, M.H., Partridge, A.J. et al. 1999. The natural history of exercise-induced anaphylaxis: survey results from a 10-year follow-up study. *J Allergy Clin Immunol*, 104, 123–7
4   Stewart, A.G. and Ewan, P.W. 1996. The incidence, aetiology and management of anaphylaxis presenting to an Accident & Emergency department. *QJM*, 89, 859–64
5   Golden, D.B. 2003. Stinging insect allergy. *Am Fam Physician*, 5, 67, 2,541–6
6   Royal College of Physicians. June 2003. *Allergy: The Unmet Need – A blueprint for better patient care*
7   Al-Muhsen, S., Clarke, A.E. and Kagan, R.S. 2003. Peanut allergy: an overview. *CMAJ*, 168, 1,279–85
8   Ewan, P.W. and Clark, A.T. 2001. Long-term prospective observational study of patients with peanut and nut allergy after participation in a management plan. *Lancet*, 357, 111–5

Chapter 5

End notes

1   Liangas, G., Morton, J.R. and Henry, R.L. 2003. Mirth-triggered asthma: Is laughter really the best medicine? *Pediatr Pulmonol*, 36, 107–12
2   Elias, J.A. 2000. Airway remodeling in asthma: Unanswered questions. *Am J Respir Crit Care Med*, 161, S168–S171
3   Skloot, G.S. 2002. Nocturnal asthma: mechanisms and management. *Mt Sinai J Med*, 69, 140–7
4   Lu, L.R., Peat, J.K. and Sullivan, C.E. 2003. Snoring in preschool children: prevalence and association with nocturnal cough and asthma. *Chest*, 124, 587–93
5   Calhoun, W.J. 2003. Nocturnal asthma. *Chest*, 123 (3 Suppl), 399S–405S
6   Morkjaroenpong, V., Rand, C.S., Butz, A.M. et al. 2002. Environmental tobacco smoke exposure and nocturnal symptoms among inner-city children with asthma. *J Allergy Clin Immunol*, 110, 147–53
7   Sheth, K.K. 2003. Activity-induced asthma. *Pediatr Clin North Am*, 50, 697–716
8   Sinha, T. and David, A.K. 2003. Recognition and management of exercise-induced bronchospasm. *Am Fam Physician*, 67, 769–74
9   Smith, E., Mahony, N., Donne, B. et al. 2002. Prevalence of obstructive airflow limitation in Irish collegiate athletes. *Ir J Med Sci*, 171, 202–5

10   Mannix, E.T., Roberts, M., Fagin, D.P. et al. 2003. The prevalence of airways hyper-responsiveness in members of an exercise training facility. *J Asthma*, 40, 349–55
11   Royal College of Physicians. June 2003. *Allergy: The Unmet Need – A blueprint for better patient care*
12   Slavin, R.G. 2003. Occupational rhinitis. *Ann Allergy Asthma Immunol*, 90 (5 Suppl 2), 2–6
13   Padoan, M., Pozzato, V., Simoni, M. et al. 2003. Long-term follow-up of toluene diisocyanate-induced asthma. *Eur Respir J*, 21, 637–40
14   Droste, J., Myny, K., Van Sprundel, M. et al. 2003. Allergic sensitization, symptoms, and lung function among bakery workers as compared with a nonexposed work population. *J Occup Environ Med*, 45, 648–55
15   Roberts, G. and Lack, G. 2003. Relevance of inhalational exposure to food allergens. *Curr Opin Allergy Clin Immunol*, 3, 211–5
16   Anees, W. 2003. Use of pulmonary function tests in the diagnosis of occupational asthma. *Ann Allergy Asthma Immunol*, 90 (5 Suppl 2), 47–51
17   Karlen, A. 1996. *Plague's Progress*. Indigo

General
Liu, Q. and Wisnewski, A.V. 2003. Recent developments in diisocyanate asthma. *Ann Allergy Asthma Immunol*, 90 (5 Suppl 2), 35–41
Roberts, G. and Lack, G. 2003. Relevance of inhalational exposure to food allergens. *Curr Opin Allergy Clin Immunol*, 3, 211–5
Vandenplas, O. and Malo, J.L. 2003. Definitions and types of work-related asthma: a nosological approach. *Eur Respir J*, 21, 706–12

Chapter 6

1   Wouters, E.F., Creutzberg, E.C. and Schols, A.M. 2002. Systemic effects in COPD. *Chest*, 121 (5 Suppl), 127S–130S
2   Sturesson, M. and Branholm, I-B. 2000. Life satisfaction in subjects with chronic obstructive pulmonary disease. *Work*, 14, 77–82
3   Barnes, P.J. 2003. Therapy of chronic obstructive pulmonary disease. *Pharmacology & Therapeutics*, 97, 87–94
4   Alsaeedi, A., Sin. D.D. and McAlister, F.A. 2002. The effects of inhaled corticosteroids in chronic obstructive pulmonary disease: a systematic review of randomised placebo-controlled trials. *Am J Med*, 113, 59–65
5   Szafranski, W., Cukier, A., Ramirez, A. et al. 2003. Efficacy and safety of budesonide/formoterol in the management of chronic obstructive pulmonary disease. *Eur Respir J*, 21, 74–81
6   British Thoracic Society, Scottish Intercollegiate Guidelines Network (SIGN). 2003. British guidelines on the management of asthma. *Thorax*, 58 (Suppl 1), i1–i194

Chapter 7

End notes

1 D'Amato, G. 2003. Therapy of allergic bronchial asthma with omalizumab – an anti-IgE monoclonal antibody. *Expert Opin Biol Ther*, 3, 371–6

2 Lafage-Proust, M.H., Boudignon, B. and Thomas, T. 2003. Glucocorticoid-induced osteoporosis: pathophysiological data and recent treatments. *Joint Bone Spine*, 70, 109–18

3 Allen, D.B., Mullen, M. and Mullen, B. 1994. A meta-analysis of the effect of oral and inhaled corticosteroids on growth. *J Allergy Clin Immunol*, 93, 967–76

4 Pedersen, S. 2002. Long-term outcomes in paediatric asthma. *Allergy*, 57 (Suppl 74), 58–74

5 Wouden, J.C., Tasche, M.J., Bernsen, R.M., Uijen, J.H., Jongste, J.C. and Ducharme, F.M. 2003. Inhaled sodium cromoglycate for asthma in children. *Cochrane Database Syst Rev* 3, CD002173

6 Barnes, P.J. 2003. Anti-leukotrienes: here to stay? *Current Opinion in Pharmacology*, 3, 1–7

7 Peters-Golden, M. 2003. Do anti-leukotriene agents inhibit asthmatic inflammation? *Clin Exp Allergy*, 33, 721–4

8 Bjermer, L., Bisgaard, H., Bousquet, J. et al. 2003. Montelukast and fluticasone compared with salmeterol and fluticasone in protecting against asthma exacerbation in adults: one year, double blind randomised comparative trial. *BMJ*, 327, 891–5

9 Rosenhall, L., Elvstrand, A., Tilling, B. et al. 2003. One-year safety and efficacy of budesonide/formoterol in a single inhaler (Symbicort Turbuhaler) for the treatment of asthma. *Respir Med*, 97, 702–8

10 Nelson, H.S., Chapman, K.R., Pyke, S.D. et al. 2003. Enhanced synergy between fluticasone propionate and salmeterol inhaled from a single inhaler versus separate inhalers. *J Allergy Clin Immunol*, 112, 29–36

General

Fozard, J.R. and Walker, C. 2003. Controversies in respiratory diseases and their management. *Current Opinion in Pharmacology*, 3, 209–11

Kercsmar, C.M. 2003. Current trends in management of pediatric asthma. *Respir Care*, 48, 194–205

Miescher, S.M. and Vogel, M. 2002. Molecular aspects of allergy. *Molecular Aspects of Medicine*, 23, 413–62

Skloot, G.S. 2002. Nocturnal asthma: mechanisms and management. *Mount Sinai J Med*, 69, 140–48

Chapter 8

1 Schultz-Larsen, F. and Hanifin, J.M. 2002. Epidemiology of atopic dermatitis. *Immunol Allergy Clin North Am*, 22, 1–24

2   Oranje, A.P. and de Waard-van der Spek, F.B. 2002. Atopic dermatitis: review 2000 to January 2001. *Curr Opin Pediatr*, 14, 410–3

3   Buske-Kirschbaum, A. and Hellhammer, D.H. 2003. Endocrine and immune responses to stress in chronic inflammatory skin disorders. *Ann NY Acad Sci*, 992, 231–40

4   Leung, D.Y.M. and Bieberc, T. 2003. Atopic dermatitis. *Lancet*, 361, 151–60

5   Burks, W. 2003. Skin manifestations of food allergy. *Pediatrics*, 111, 1,617–24

6   Nola, I., Kostovic, K., Kotrulja, L. et al. 2003. The use of emollients as sophisticated therapy in dermatology. *Acta Dermatovenerol Croat*, 11, 80–7

7   *Oral antihistamines for allergic disorders*. Drug and Therapeutics Bulletin, Vol 40, No 8, Aug 2002

8   *Topical steroids for atopic dermatitis in primary care*. Drug and Therapeutics Bulletin, Vol 41, No 1, Jan 2003

9   *Topical tacrolimus – a role in atopic dermatitis?*. Drug and Therapeutics Bulletin, Vol 40, No 10, Oct 2002

10 The Royal College of Physicians. June 2003. *Allergy: The Unmet Need – A blueprint for better patient care*

11 Meyer, J.D., Chen, Y., Holt, D.L., et al. 2000. Occupational contact dermatitis in the UK: a surveillance report from EPIDERM and OPRA. *Occup Med*, 50, 265–73

12 Rietschel, R.L. 1997. Occupational contact dermatitis. *Lancet*, 349, 1,093–5

13 Fregert, S. 1975. Occupational dermatitis in a 10-year material. *Contact Dermatitis*, 1, 96–107

Chapter 9

End notes

1   Royal College of Physicians. June 2003. *Allergy: The Unmet Need – A blueprint for better patient care*

2   Salib, R.J., Drake-Lee, A. and Howarth, P.H. 2003. Allergic rhinitis: past, present and the future. *Clin Otolaryngol*, 28, 291–303

3   Berger, W.E. 2003. Overview of allergic rhinitis. *Ann Allergy Asthma Immunol*, 90 (6 Suppl 3), 7–12

4   Rucci, L., Bocciolini, C. and Casucci, A. 2003. Nasal polyposis: microsurgical ethmoidectomy and interruption of autonomic innervation vs conventional surgery. *Acta Otorhinolaryngol Ital*, 23, 26–32

5   Crown, W.H., Olufade, A., Smith, M.W. et al. 2003. Seasonal versus perennial allergic rhinitis: drug and medical resource use patterns. *Value Health*, 6, 448–56

6   Bousquet, J., Vignola, A.M. and Demoly, P. 2003. Links between rhinitis and asthma. *Allergy*, 58, 691–706

7   Sheikh, A. and Hurwitz, B. 2003. House dust mite avoidance measures for perennial allergic rhinitis: a systematic review of efficacy. *Br J Gen Pract*, 53, 318–22

8   Terreehorst, I., Hak, E., Oosting, A.J. et al. 2003. Evaluation of impermeable covers for bedding in patients with allergic rhinitis. *N Engl J Med*, 349, 237–46

9   Hughes, K., Glass, C., Ripchinski, M. et al. 2003. Efficacy of the topical nasal steroid budesonide on improving sleep and daytime somnolence in patients with perennial allergic rhinitis. *Allergy*, 58, 380–5

10 Moller, C., Ahlstrom, H., Henricson, K.A. et al. 2003. Safety of nasal budesonide in the long-term treatment of children with perennial rhinitis. *Clin Exp Allergy*, 33, 816–22

11 Weiner, J.M., Abramson, M.J., Puy, R.M. et al. 1998. Intranasal corticosteroids versus oral H1 receptor antagonists in allergic rhinitis: systematic review of randomised controlled trials. *BMJ*, 317, 1,624–9

12 Lin, H.C., Lin, P.W., Su, C.Y. et al. 2003. Radiofrequency for the treatment of allergic rhinitis refractory to medical therapy. *Laryngoscope*, 113, 673–8

General

Lee, N.P. and Arriola, E.R. 1999. How to treat allergic rhinitis. *West J Med*, 171, 31–4

Linneberg, A., Henrik Nielsen, N., Frøeund, L. et al. 2002. The link between allergic rhinitis and allergic asthma: a prospective population-based study. The Copenhagen Allergy Study. *Allergy*, 57, 1,048–52

Chapter 10

End notes

1   Church, M.K. and McGill, J.I. 2002. Human ocular mast cells. *Curr Opin Allergy Clin Immunol*, 2, 419–22

2   Strauss, E.C. and Foster, C.S. 2002. Atopic ocular disease. *Ophthalmol Clin North Am*, 15, 1–5

3   Stapleton, F., Stretton, S., Sankaridurg, P.R. et al. 2003. Hypersensitivity responses and contact lens wear. *Contact Lens & Anterior Eye*, 26, 57–69

4   Wuthrich, B., Brignoli, R., Canevascini, M. et al. 1998. Epidemiological survey in hay fever patients: symptom prevalence and severity and influence on patient management. *Schweiz Med Wochenschr*, 128, 139–43

5   Austin, J.B., Kaur, B., Anderson, H.R. et al. 1999. Hay fever, eczema, and wheeze: a nationwide UK study (ISAAC, international study of asthma and allergies in childhood), *Arch Dis Child*; 81, 225–30

6   Howarth, P. 2002. Antihistamines in rhinoconjunctivitis. *Clin Allergy Immunol*, 17, 179–220

7   Alexander, M., Allegro, S. and Hicks, A. 2001. Nedocromil sodium in golfers with seasonal allergic conjunctivitis, *Adv Ther*, 18, 195–204

8   Nazarov, O., Petzold, U., Haase, H. et al. 2003. Azelastine eye drops in the treatment of perennial allergic conjunctivitis, *Arzneimittelforschung*, 53, 167–73

9   Martin, A.P., Urrets-Zavalia, J., Berra, A. et al. 2003. The effect of ketotifen on inflammatory markers in allergic conjunctivitis: an open, uncontrolled study. *BMC Ophthalmology*, 3, 2 (www.biomedcentral.com/1471-2415/3/2)

10 Rajan, T.V., Tennen, H., Lindquist, R.L., et al. 2002. Effect of ingestion of honey on symptoms of rhinoconjunctivitis. *Ann Allergy Asthma Immunol,* 88, 198–203

General

Bisca, M. 1997. Current therapy of allergic conjunctivitis. *Current Therapeutic Research*, 58, 828–41

Friedlaender, M.H. 1995. A review of the causes and treatment of bacterial and allergic conjunctivitis. *Clinical Therapeutics*, 17, 800–10

Chapter 11

End notes

1   *Nut Allergies*, Health Which?, Dec 1997, pp 158–9

2   Al-Muhsen, S., Clarke, A.E. and Kagan, R.S. 2003. Peanut allergy: an overview. *CMAJ*, 168, 1,279–85

3   Wood, R.A. 2003. The natural history of food allergy. *Pediatrics*, 111, 1,631–7

4   Tariq, S.M., Stevens, M., Matthews, S. et al. 1996. Cohort study of peanut and tree nut sensitisation by age of 4 years. *BMJ*, 313, 514–7

5   Grundy, J., Matthews, S., Bateman, B. et al. 2002. Rising prevalence of allergy to peanut in children: Data from 2 sequential cohorts. *J Allergy Clin Immunol*, 110, 784–9

6   Royal College of Physicians. June 2003. *Allergy: The Unmet Need – A blue-print for better patient care*

7   *Good or Bad?*, Health Which?, Feb 2003, p 31

8   Roberts, G. and Lack, G. 2003. Relevance of inhalational exposure to food allergens. *Curr Opin Allergy Clin Immunol*, 3, 211–5

9   Roberts, G., Patel, N., Levi-Schaffer, F. et al. 2003. Food allergy as a risk factor for life-threatening asthma in childhood: a case-controlled study. *J Allergy Clin Immunol*, 112, 168–74

10 Ewan, P.W. and Clark, A.T. 2001. Long-term prospective observational study of patients with peanut and nut allergy after participation in a management plan. *Lancet*, 357, 111–5

11 Mowat, A.M. 2003. Coeliac disease – a meeting point for genetics, immunology, and protein chemistry. *Lancet*, 361, 1,290–2

12 Al Attas, R.A. 2002. How common is celiac disease in eastern Saudi Arabia? *Annals of Saudi Medicine*, 22, 315–9

13   Catassi, C, Fornaroli F. and Fasano, A. 2002. Celiac disease: From basic immunology to bedside practice. *Clinical and Applied Immunology Reviews*, 3, 61–71

14   Teuber, S.S. and Porch-Curren, C. 2003. Unproved diagnostic and therapeutic approaches to food allergy and intolerance. *Curr Opin Allergy Clin Immunol*, 3, 217–21

15   Osterballe, M. and Bindslev-Jensen, C. 2003. Threshold levels in food challenge and specific IgE in patients with egg allergy: is there a relationship? *J Allergy Clin Immunol*, 112, 196–201

16   Crespo, J.F., Rodriguez, J., James, J.M. et al. 2002. Reactivity to potential cross-reactive foods in fruit-allergic patients: implications for prescribing food avoidance. *Allergy*, 57, 946–49

17   *GM & Food Allergies*, Health Which?, June 2002, pp 16–9

General

Bahna, S.L. 2003. Clinical expressions of food allergy. *Ann Allergy Asthma Immunol*, 90 (6 Suppl 3), 41–4

Hubbard, S. 2003. Nutrition and food allergies: the dietician's role. *Ann Allergy Asthma Immunol*, 90 (6 Suppl 3), 115–6

Chapter 12

End notes

1   Riedl, M.A. and Casillas, A.M. 2003. Adverse drug reactions: types and treatment options. *Am Fam Physician*, 68, 1,781

2   Vervloet, D. and Durham, S. 1998. Adverse reactions to drugs. *BMJ*, 316, 1,511–4

3   Royal College of Physicians. June 2003. *Allergy: The Unmet Need – A blueprint for better patient care*

4   Nigen, S., Knowles, S.R. and Shear, N.H. 2003. Drug eruptions: approaching the diagnosis of drug-induced skin diseases. *J Drugs Dermatol*, 2, 278–99

5   Pichler, W.J. 2003. Delayed drug hypersensitivity reactions. *Ann Intern Med*, 139, 683–93

6   Wright, A.J. 1999. The Penicillins. *Mayo Clin Proc*, 74, 290–307

7   Miller, E.L. 2002. The penicillins: A review and update. *J Midwifery Women's Health*, 47, 426–34

8   Salkind, A.R., Cuddy, P.G., Foxworth, J.W. 2001. Is this patient allergic to penicillin? An evidence-based analysis of the likelihood of penicillin allergy. *JAMA*, 285, 2,498–505

9   Rang, H.P., Dale, M.M. and Ritter, J.M. 1999. *Pharmacology*. Churchill Livingstone

General

Boelsterli, U.A. 2003. *Mechanistic Toxicology.* Taylor & Francis

Chapter 13

1   Steurer-Stey, C., Russi, E.W. and Steurer, J. 2002. Complementary and alternative medicine in asthma – do they work? A summary and appraisal of published evidence. *Swiss Med Wkly*, 132, 338–44

2   Kay, A.B. and Lessof, M.H. 1992. Allergy. Conventional and alternative concepts. A report of the Royal College of Physicians Committee on Clinical Immunology and Allergy. *Clin Exp Allergy*, 22 (Suppl 3), 1–44

3   Shapiro, A.K. and Shapiro, E. 1997. *The Powerful Placebo.* The John Hopkins University Press

4   Niggemann, B. and Grüber, C. 2003. Side-effects of complementary and alternative medicine. *Allergy*, 58, 707–16

5   Royal College of Physicians. June 2003. *Allergy: The Unmet Need – A blueprint for better patient care*

6   Huntley, A., White, A.R. and Ernst, E. 2002. Relaxation therapies for asthma: a systematic review. *Thorax*, 57, 127–31

7   Lane, D.J. and Lane, T.V. 1991. Alternative and complementary medicine for asthma. *Thorax*, 46, 787–97

8   Dennis, J. 2000. Alexander technique for chronic asthma. *Cochrane Database Syst Rev*, 2, CD000995

9   Cooper, S., Oborne, J., Newton, S., et al. 2003. Effect of two breathing exercises (Buteyko and pranayama) in asthma: a randomised controlled trial. *Thorax*, 58, 674–9

10 Bowler, S.D., Green, A. and Mitchell, C.A. 1998. Buteyko breathing techniques in asthma: a blinded randomised controlled trial. *Med J Aust*, 169, 575–8

11 Schulman, S. 2003. Addressing the potential risks associated with ephedra use: a review of recent efforts. *Public Health Rep*, 118, 487–92

12 Worm, M. 2002. Novel therapies for atopic eczema. *Current Opinion in Investigational Drugs*, 3 (11), 1,596–603

13 *Steroids in Herbal Medicines*, Which?, May 2001, p 13 (see also *Inside Story*, Which?, April 2003, p 5)

14 Fung, A.Y., Look, P.C., Chong, L.Y., et al. 1999. A controlled trial of traditional Chinese herbal medicine in Chinese patients with recalcitrant atopic dermatitis. *Int J Dermatol*, 38, 387–92

15 Armstrong, N.C. and Ernst, E. 1999. The treatment of eczema with Chinese herbs: a systematic review of randomized clinical trials. *Br J Clin Pharmacol*, 48, 262–4

16 Latchman, Y., Banerjee, P., Poulter, L.W. et al. 1996. Association of immunological changes with clinical efficacy in atopic eczema patients treated with traditional Chinese herbal therapy (Zemaphyte). *Int Arch Allergy Immunol*, 109, 243–9

17 *Alternative Update*, Health Which?, June 2002, p 36

18 Reilly, D.T., Taylor, M.A., McSharry, C. et al. 1986. Is homoeopathy a placebo response? Controlled trial of homoeopathic potency, with pollen in hayfever as model. *Lancet*, ii, 881–6

19 Taylor, M.A., Reilly, D., Llewellyn-Jones, R.H. et al. 2000. Randomised controlled trial of homoeopathy versus placebo in perennial allergic rhinitis with overview of four trial series. *BMJ*, 321, 471–6

20 Reilly, D.T., Taylor, M.A., Beattie, N.G.M. et al. 1994. Is evidence for homoeopathy reproducible? *Lancet*, 344, 1,601–6

21 White, A., Slade, P., Hunt, C., et al. 2003. Individualised homeopathy as an adjunct in the treatment of childhood asthma: a randomised placebo controlled trial. *Thorax*, 58, 317–21

22 Lewith, G.T., Watkins, A.D., Hyland, M.E. et al. 2002. Use of ultramolecular potencies of allergen to treat asthmatic people allergic to house dust mite: double blind randomised controlled clinical trial. *BMJ*, 324, 520

23 Barnett, H. 2002. *The Which? Guide to Complementary Therapies*. Which? Books

24 Hackman, R.M., Stern, J.S. and Gershwin, M.E. 2000. Hypnosis and asthma: a critical review. *J Asthma*, 37, 1–15

25 Shenefelt, P.D. 2003. Biofeedback, cognitive-behavioural methods, and hypnosis in dermatology: Is it all in your mind? *Dermatol Ther*, 16 (2), 114–22

26 Wilson, A.F., Honsberger. R., Chiu. J.T., et al. 1975. Transcendental meditation and asthma. *Respiration*, 32, 74–80

27 Manocha, R., Marks, G.B., Kenchington, P., et al. 2002. Sahaja yoga in the management of moderate to severe asthma: a randomised controlled trial. *Thorax*, 57, 110–5

28 Nagarathna, R. and Nagendra, H.R. 1985. Yoga for bronchial asthma: a controlled study. *BMJ*, 291, 1,077–9

29 Vedanthan, P.K., Kesavalu, L.N., Murthy, K.C. et al. 1998. Clinical study of yoga techniques in university students with asthma: a controlled study. *Allergy Asthma Proc*, 19, 3–9

30 *Stretched to the Limit*, Health Which?, August 2003, pp 10–3

Further reading

Barnett, H. 2002. *The Which? Guide to Complementary Therapies.* Which? Books

Brooks, P. and Brewer, Dr S. (Introduction). 2001. *The* Daily Telegraph *Complete Guide to Allergies.* Constable and Robinson

Brostoff, J. and Gamlin, L. 1999. *The Complete Guide to Asthma.* Bloomsbury

Brostoff, J. and Gamlin, L. 1998. *The Complete Guide to Food Allergy and Intolerance.* Bloomsbury

Grant, R. 2003. *Which? Medicine.* Which? Books

Greener, M. 2002. *The Which? Guide to Managing Stress.* Which? Books

Greer, R. 2001. *Easy Wheat, Egg, and Milk-Free Cooking.* Thorsons

Levy, S., Hilton, M. and Barnes, G. 2000. *Asthma at Your Fingertips.* Class Publishing

Savill, A. 2000. *The Gluten, Wheat and Dairy Free Cookbook.* Thorsons

Wright, T. and Clarke, G. 2001. *Food Allergies: Enjoying Life with a Severe Food Allergy.* Class Publishing

Addresses and websites

Acupuncture Association of Chartered Physiotherapists
AACP Secretariat
Portcullis
Castle Street
Mere
Wiltshire BA12 6JE
Tel: (01747) 861151
Fax: (01747) 861717
Email: aacpsecretariat@btinternet.com
Website: www.aacp.uk.com

Allergy UK
Deepdene House
30 Bellegrove Road
Welling
Kent DA16 3PY
Helpline: 020-8303 8583
Fax: 020-8303 8792
Email: info@allergyuk.org
Website: www.allergyuk.org

Anaphylaxis Campaign
PO Box 275
Farnborough
Hampshire GU14 6SX
Helpline: (01252) 542029
Fax: (01252) 377140
Email: info@anaphylaxis.org.uk
Website: www.anaphylaxis.org.uk

Arthritis Care
18 Stephenson Way
London NW1 2HD
Helpline: (0808) 800 4050 *12pm–4pm Mon–Fri*
Source helpline: (0808) 808 2000 *10am–2pm Mon–Fri*
(for young people with arthritis)
Tel: 020-7380 6500
Fax: 020-7380 6505
Email: helplines@arthritiscare.org.uk; thesource@arthritiscare.org.uk
Website: www.arthritiscare.org.uk

Arthritis Research Campaign
PO Box 177
Chesterfield
Derbyshire S41 7TQ
Tel: (01246) 558033
Website: www.arc.org.uk

British Acupuncture Council (BAcC)
63 Jeddo Road
London W12 9HQ
Tel: 020-8735 0400
Fax: 020-8735 0404
Email: info@acupuncture.org.uk
Website: www.acupuncture.org.uk

British Medical Acupuncture Society
BMAS House
3 Winnington Court
Northwich
Cheshire CW8 1AQ
Tel: (01606) 786782
Fax: (01606) 786783
Email: admin@medical-acupuncture.org.uk
Website: www.medical-acupuncture.co.uk

British Society for Allergy and Clinical Immunology (BSACI)
17 Doughty Street
LondonWC1 2LN
Tel: 020-7404 0278
Email: info@bsaci.org
Website: www.bsaci.org

British Thoracic Society
17 Doughty Street
London WC1N 2PL
Tel: 020-7831 8778
Fax: 020-7831 8766
Email: bts@brit-thoracic.org.uk
Website: www.brit-thoracic.org.uk

British Wheel of Yoga
25 Jermyn Street
Sleaford
Lincolnshire NG34 7RU
Tel: (01529) 306851
Fax: (01529) 303233
Email: office@bwy.org.uk
Website: www.bwy.org.uk

Buddhist Society UK
58 Eccleston Square
London SW1V 1PH
Tel: 020-7834 5858
Fax: 020-7976 5238
Email: info@thebuddhistsociety.org.uk
Website: www.thebuddhistsociety.org.uk

Central Register of Advanced Hypnotherapists (CRAH)
PO Box 14526
London N4 2WG
Tel: 020-7354 9938
Website: www.n-shap-ericksonian.co.uk/crah.htm
Send an A5 SAE for leaflets and further information

Coeliac UK
PO Box 220
Suite 1–3
First Floor
Octagon Court
High Wycombe
Bucks HP11 2HY
Tel: (01494) 437278
Fax: (01494) 474349
Email: admin@coeliac.co.uk
Website: www.coeliac.co.uk

Digestive Disorders Foundation
PO Box 251
Edgware
Middlesex HA8 6HG
Website: www.digestivedisorders.org.uk
For information and leaflets, send an SAE and detail what information you require

Eczema Scotland
84 West Main Street
Broxburn
West Lothian
Tel: (01506) 852033

Ethics and Anti-doping Directorate
Drug Information Database
Tel: (0800) 528 0004
Website: www.uksport.gov.uk/did

**European Federation of Allergy and Airways Diseases
Patients' Association**
Avenue Louise 327
1050 Brussels
Belgium
Tel: +32 2 646 9945
Website: www.efanet.org

Faculty of Homeopathy
Hahnemann House
29 Park Street West
Luton
Bedfordshire LU1 3BE
Tel: (08704) 443950
Fax: (08704) 443960
Email: info@trusthomeopathy.org
Website: www.trusthomeopathy.org

HSE Information Services
Caerphilly Business Park
Caerphilly CF83 3GG
Tel: (08701) 545500
Fax: 029-2085 9260
Email: hseinformationservices@natbrit.com
Website: www.hse.gov.uk

Latex Allergy Support Group
PO Box 27
Filey YO14 9YH
Helpline: (07071) 225838
Email: latexallergyfree@hotmail.com
Website: www.lasg.co.uk

MedicAlert Foundation
1 Bridge Wharf
156 Caledonian Road
London N1 9UU
Tel: 020-7833 3034
Fax: 020-7278 0647
Email: info@medicalert.org.uk
Website: www.medicalert.org.uk

National Asthma Campaign
Providence House
Providence Place
London N1 0NT
Nurses' Advice Helpline: (08457) 010203
Email: enquiries@asthma.org.uk
Website: www.asthma.org.uk

National Asthma Campaign Scotland
2a North Charlotte Street
Edinburgh EH2 4HR
Tel: (0131) 226 2544
Fax: (0131) 226 2401
Email: enquiries@asthma.org.uk
Website: www.asthma.org.uk

National Eczema Society
Hill House
Highgate Hill
London N19 5NA
Helpline: (0870) 241 3604
Tel: 020-7281 3553
Fax: 020-7281 6395
Email: helpline@eczema.org
Website: www.eczema.org

National Institute of Medical Herbalists (NIMH)
56 Longbrook Street
Exeter EX4 6AH
Tel: (01392) 426022
Fax: (01392) 498963
Email: nimh@ukexeter.freeserve.co.uk
Website: www.nimh.org.uk

National Pollen Research Unit
University College Worcester
Henwick Grove
Worcester WR2 6AJ
Website: http://pollenuk.worc.ac.uk

National Register of Hypnotherapists and Psychotherapists
Suite B
12 Cross Street
Nelson BB9 7EN
Tel: (01282) 716839
Fax: (01282) 698633
Email: nrhp@btconnect.com
Website: www.nrhp.co.uk

Register of Chinese Herbal Medicine
Office 5
Ferndale Business Centre
1 Exeter Street
Norwich NR2 4QB
Tel: (01603) 623994
Fax: (01603) 667557
Email: herbmed@rchm.co.uk
Website: www.rchm.co.uk
The RCHM can direct you to your nearest RCHM member for help and advice, but cannot answer medical queries

Society of Homeopaths
11 Brookfield
Duncan Close
Moulton Park
Northampton NN3 6WL
Tel: (0845) 450 6611
Fax: (0845) 450 6622
Email: info@homeopathy-soh.org
Website: www.homeopathy-soh.org

Society of Teachers of the Alexander Technique (STAT)
First Floor
Linton House
39–51 Highgate Road
London NW5 1RS
Tel: (0845) 230 7828
Fax: 020-7482 5435
Email: enquiries@stat.org.uk
Website: www.stat.org.uk

Transcendental Meditation
Tel: (08705) 143733 *10am–5pm, Mon–Fri*
Website: www.transcendental-meditation.org.uk
Further information and details of your local centre can be found on the website or by telephoning the above number

Yoga for Health Foundation
Ickwell Bury
Biggleswade
Bedfordshire SG18 9EF
Tel: (01767) 627271
Fax: (01767) 627266
Email: admin@yogaforhealthfoundation.co.uk
Website: www.yogaforhealthfoundation.co.uk

Which? Books
PO Box 44
Hertford SG14 1SH
Tel: (0800) 252100
Email: books@which.co.uk
Website: www.which.net.

Websites

There is a plethora of websites covering asthma and allergies. Some of the more reputable are listed below.

UK sites
Action Against Allergy: www.actionagainstallergy.co.uk
Allergic Diseases: www.allergicdiseases.co.uk
Asthma and Allergy Information and Research:
    www.users.globalnet.co.uk/~aair
British Lung Foundation: www.britishlungfoundation.org
General Practice Airways Group: www.gpiag.org

Health & Safety Executive (occupational asthma):
   www.hse.gov.uk/asthma
Lung and Asthma Information Agency:
   www.sghms.ac.uk/depts/laia/laia.htm
Midlands Asthma & Allergy Research Association: www.maara.org
Sinus News: www.sinusnews.com (covers sinusitis, allergies and asthma)
Which? Online: www.which.net
   Which? Online is a subscription service with a free three-month trial period

International sites
The following sites may also offer some valuable advice. But remember that the drugs and doses suggested on these sites may not be available in the UK.

Allergy, Asthma and Immunology online: http://allergy.mcg.edu/
American Academy of Allergy, Asthma and Immunology: www.aaaai.org
University of Michigan's asthma site: www.med.umich.edu/wheas

Index

SCOTTISH BORDERS COUNCIL

LIBRARY &
INFORMATION SERVICES